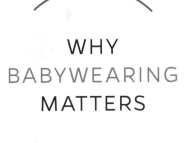

WHY
BABYWEARING
MATTERS

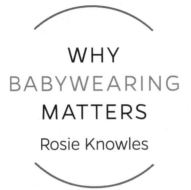

WHY BABYWEARING MATTERS

Rosie Knowles

pinter
&
martin

Why Babywearing Matters (Pinter & Martin Why It Matters 5)

First published by Pinter & Martin Ltd 2016

ISBN 978-1-78066-535-1

Also available as an ebook

Pinter & Martin Why It Matters ISSN 2056-8567

Series editor: Susan Last
Index: Helen Bilton
Design: Rebecca Longworth
Proofreader: Debbie Kennett

The publishers and the author cannot accept responsibility for any damage incurred as a result of using any of the equipment mentioned or following any of the methods contained in this work. If you are unsure of the suitability of any of the equipment or methods in this book, it is advisable to consult a healthcare practitioner or professional.

In the interests of anonymity, some names have been changed.

British Library Cataloguing-in-Publication Data
A catalogue record for this book is available from the British Library.

Set in Minion

Printed and bound in the UK by Ashford Colour Press Ltd, Gosport, Hampshire

This book has been printed on paper that is sourced and harvested from sustainable forests and is FSC accredited.

Pinter & Martin Ltd
6 Effra Parade
London SW2 1PS

pinterandmartin.com

Contents

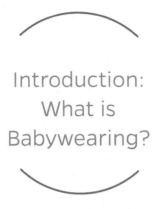

Introduction: What is Babywearing?

Children have been carried in their parents' arms from the very beginning of the human story; it is a practice that transcends evolution, history, geography, society and culture. A baby's natural habitat is his mother's body; she is the source of love, nourishment, safety and warmth.

Responding to a child's cry is an instinctive, natural activity. The sound of such an innocent need tugs at the heartstrings of a parent, especially the mother who carried and birthed her baby, and provokes an intense emotional desire to meet that need. Many adults and older children also feel this urge to respond to an infant's request for interaction; human contact with other humans is vital to emotional and physical health and is a normal and essential part of development.

Infants and children who grow up in communities where they are deeply loved and respected have the advantage of feeling secure and being certain of their own value. One of the best ways of providing this sense of love and security to a small child is to carry them in arms, right from birth.

A baby who has spent all his life growing in the womb, first floating in water and then gently compressed by uterine walls, will find the sensation of freedom and open space in the outside world enormously different. Limbs that have been limited are suddenly free to stretch wide, darkness has turned to light, the muffled gentle rhythmic sounds of the mother's body have been replaced by loud, unfamiliar noises or deep silence, constant gentle motion has turned into complete stillness or sudden liftings into nothingness. The 'fourth trimester' – the first few months of a child's life in the outside world – is all about gentle transitioning from the peace and stability of the womb towards active involvement in a new world. A newborn needs to be supported to gain skills and strength at a steady, individual pace from the security of an unshakeable foundation and a place of comfort and familiarity.

In the medical world, there is a growing consensus about the enormous value of 'kangaroo care'. It has long been known that babies born early and very small can survive against the odds if they are placed skin-to-skin against their mother's chest, inside a shirt, as if in a kangaroo pouch. This stabilises the baby's heart and respiratory rates, and helps them modulate their temperature. Kangaroo care, compared to standard hospital care, reduces infection, hypothermia, severe illness, respiratory tract disease and the length of hospital stay. Successful breastfeeding is more likely to be established. It is clear that skin-to-skin contact is of huge benefit, and many birth practitioners encourage instant passing of the newly born baby on to the mother's chest, before any washing or cord cutting. Hospitals around the world are beginning to introduce kangaroo care as standard practice in special care baby units wherever possible. Yet it is not only those born early or sick who benefit; close contact is just as vital for healthy term babies.

The skin is the largest and most sensitive organ in the body and is readily and easily accessible; it provides an enormous amount of sensory information to the growing brain. The sense of touch is the most powerful of the six senses, and loving touch is vital to healthy physiological and psychological growth. Babies born without sight, hearing or a sense of smell need not be too disadvantaged in their future development, but babies deprived of touch and emotional support fail to thrive; this is the cornerstone of attachment theory.

Attachment (in the evolutionary sense) is the deep and enduring emotional bond that connects one person to another across time and space; a 'lasting psychological connectedness between human beings.'[1] There is a growing body of convincing observational and neurobiological evidence that attachment really matters; it is the bedrock for emotional and physical health, and for children is the springboard to confident independence later in life. Having a strong, reliable, trustworthy set of loving, intimate relationships allows children to thrive; when this is missing, problems arise that affect wider society. Consistent, appropriate loving touch really does matter.

Carrying a baby close to the chest provides this loving touch and offers a great sense of familiarity and normality for a newborn. They hear the muffled thump of a heartbeat and the rhythm of regular breathing that they are used to, gentle pressure from cradling arms provides security and a mother's scent means safety and nourishment. No wonder babies need to be carried and thrive when they are!

Cultures the world over have long realised the advantages of using a cloth carrier to keep babies close, while having hands free to do the daily work of living. Many traditional communities help new parents to care for their children in the early weeks by sharing their normal workload, a practice that our own society used to employ (lying-in) until relatively recently. But the time will come when new parents need to re-enter their societies. Using a sling to bind still-young children to their bodies allows the nurturing bond to be protected while life goes on, while fields are tilled or water is collected, or while going about household tasks, or reconnecting when returning from work.

In recent years the practice of using some form of sling or carrier to hold a baby securely against a caregiver's body has become known in many circles as 'babywearing'. This term was first coined by paediatrician Dr William Sears in the 1980s to describe the act of holding a child so close it is almost as if they were being worn in clothing. As his website explains:

'Babywearing means changing your mindset of what babies are really like. New parents often envision babies as lying quietly in a crib, gazing passively at dangling mobiles and picked up and carried only to be fed and played with and then put down. You may think that 'up' periods are just dutiful intervals to quiet your baby long enough to put him down again. Babywearing reverses this view. Carry your baby in a sling many hours a day, and then put her down for sleep times and tend to your personal needs.'[2]

In short, babies are dependent little souls who rely on their parents for every need. Their means of communication are limited – they can only utter noises and cries – and mostly their needs are simple: to be close, to be loved, to be fed, to be warm, clean and dry, to be listened to and to be valued. Carrying your child, interacting deeply with them, being in tune with them and responsive to their expressed needs is vital: it gives a sense of belonging, of being rooted, of having a place in the world. Such a strong foundation allows human infants to grow into secure, confident children and loving, caring adults capable of positive relationships, which leads to a more stable society.

While there is a strong evidence base for the value of skin-to-skin contact in premature infants and newborns, and kangaroo care is well established in many hospitals as a result, there is a lack of robust, large-scale studies of baby carriers and their use beyond the neonatal unit. This means that some healthcare professionals are wary about recommending babywearing. However, a lack of formal research doesn't necessarily mean something is ineffective or useless, particularly in the context of a practice that has been common across much of human history. Small studies can be suggestive of potential benefits, and as carrying in arms is a simple, easily available tool parents can use in the care of their children, it should be recommended more often. Baby carriers, when used safely, have great potential to make the lives of parents easier, as well as providing the close contact that children thrive on. I don't believe that the lack of studies should prevent the widespread use and promotion of carrying in arms or safely in a sling by those involved with families in the early years of parenting. I believe that funding for proper research and large-scale studies into the positive effects of carrying will benefit our society as a whole.

This book explores the history of carrying children across human evolution and cultures, and examines why it matters so much, especially in the world we find ourselves living in today. We'll find out why carrying a child is vital to developing relationships, and the role it plays in nurturing and feeding. We'll discuss why carrying is in decline, and look at how babywearing can make a difference to families experiencing the challenges of living in our modern society with its pressures and expectations. We'll see how carrying can help those struggling with depression, and how society as a whole can benefit from keeping children close. We will also learn how to carry a child safely and comfortably, the basics of good positioning in arms and in a sling, and look at the most common types of carrier. We'll deal with some common concerns about slings, and look at how to get specialist help with more complex situations, as well as local advice and support.

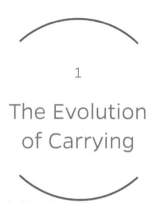

1

The Evolution
of Carrying

We can learn a lot about carrying babies from studying the natural world. The practice of carrying infants close to a parent's body can be observed across our evolutionary history, especially among the primates. The great apes, to which humans are most closely related, carry their babies underneath their bodies or on their backs when they move around. Most primate infants, when they are born, are not yet able to move around independently in the manner of their species, so they are adapted to hold on to the fur of their mother's belly with their hands and feet from birth. Such infants are classified as 'active clinging young'; they can hold on to their mothers independently and move with her, rather than sleeping in a nest, huddled in a litter, to which the mother returns. It is here, firmly attached to their parent for lengthy periods, that clinging infants are able to complete their physiological and neurological development into independent animals. Their mother's body is where they learn the skills they need, and she remains a 'safe place', a haven to flee to when danger threatens.[1]

As humans have evolved from our great ape ancestors,

their pelvises have changed and altered over time. A human pelvis is wider, and has changed in alignment to allow us to stand upright and walk unsupported on two legs.

Bipedalism allowed australopithecines (a species between apes and hominins, the famous 'Lucy') to move faster on two legs, and their hands became less like feet, developing into incredibly useful tools. Hands that could be used for carrying and throwing were a major evolutionary advantage. However, the change in the skeletal anatomy of the pelvis made it harder for the infant australopithecine's head to pass through the mother's pelvic girdle at birth, and as hominin brains grew larger, the 'obstetrical dilemma'[2] developed. Efficient bipedal locomotion requires a narrower, more lightweight pelvis with a smaller birth canal, but the increasing size of the brain with growing intelligence means the skull has to increase in size.

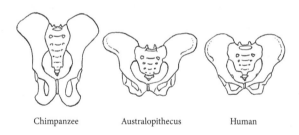

Chimpanzee   Australopithecus   Human

Humans have solved this problem by evolving the maternal pelvis further; the pelvic outlet has widened to allow the passage of the skull, and the iliac crests have altered to their current supportive shape. The birth process itself has also adapted: human babies' bodies rotate during delivery so that the cranium and shoulders can pass through the birth canal.[3] Furthermore, the overall size of the human infant at birth (with its large cranium) is nearly twice as large in relation to its mother's weight as would be expected for another similarly sized primate. After about nine months of pregnancy, the energetic demands of the growing human baby begin to surpass the mother's ability to fuel continued growth.[4] Human babies are therefore born at an earlier stage of their development than their primate counterparts, and their brains are considerably less developed at birth (25–30 per cent, compared to nearer 50 per cent for primate infants[5,6]).

As a result, human babies have one of the longest 'exterogestation' periods of any species: they are known as 'altricial' young, born helpless and dependent on their caregivers. It takes many months for human babies to be able to walk, talk and feed themselves; they need adults for safety, provision of food, warmth and emotional development.

The earliest human ancestors differed further from the great apes when they began to lose their fur. The infants of *Australopithecus* and subsequent hominins would not have been able to cling on to their relatively hairless mothers with their changed anatomy. Legs and feet that need to be fully weight-bearing and able to walk upright are very different from those that need to grip and climb trees. Our evolutionary origins are still visible in human babies; consider the 'primitive reflexes' of the palmar grasp of the palms (a gripping motion of the hands) and the Moro reflex (the startle reaction). These reflexes are believed to be remnants of human evolutionary history, designed to help the baby cling to the mother while being carried, and to encourage the regaining of a firm hold if balance was lost.[7]

That the grasp reflex in infants has persisted long beyond the loss of hair suggests that it still serves a useful purpose. It is thought that human babies will still cling on instinctively, and will continue to do so if their inbuilt reflexes are encouraged rather than suppressed by being put down at every opportunity.

Human newborn babies cling to their mothers by curling themselves into her body to make carrying easy; their curved spines facilitate this. When you pick up a newborn you will often see them tuck their legs into a squatting position to be carried on the front or the shoulder, and they often sleep like this too.

In *A Baby Wants to Be Carried*[8] Dr Evelin Kirkilionis argues convincingly that as the skeletons and pelvic alignment of hominins adapted to walk upright and allow the passage of large skulls through the birth canal, the carrying of older infants on the hip also became possible. A wider pelvis with protruding iliac bones that arch outwards, combined with a narrower waist, creates a distinct shape that is not seen in apes or early hominins. This waist to hip curve means that a baby can 'ride' astride his mother, and she can distribute most of her child's weight through her own major weight-bearing axes (the pelvis and long bones of the leg).

This is an 'exaptation': a trait that originally evolved for one purpose, but has come to serve another that also encourages the advance of that species. Dr Kirkilionis suggests that this exaptation of the spread-squat position of our ape ancestors with feet angled towards each other, into the perching astride and gripping action of the human baby, meant that the human race could continue to evolve and thrive as a bipedal upright species. She believes this is why human babies have not lost their primitive reflexes and why they continue to demonstrate the commonly-observed knees up and spread-apart (M-shape) posture when lying down and when picked up. As the young baby grows, his hip opening angle becomes wider and wider, to 'fit' around his mother's hip/waist region and grip her sides with his thighs. This allows the heavier child to cling on, helping his mother to support him while the family is on the move, improving the chances of survival.

Furthermore, the natural spread-squat position that an

infant adopts when carried astride the hip is the ideal leg position for the healthy development of their own hip joint for later walking. Studies show that babies, when held simply by an arm around their backs and not in a sling, abducted their legs an average of 45 degrees from the midline (making the total angle between knee to groin to opposite knee about 90 degrees), and raised their knees upwards to bend the hip to between 90 and 120 degrees. These angles are almost identical to those recommended by orthopaedic specialists to encourage the correct development of dysplastic (shallow) hip sockets. Dr Kirkilionis suggests that the spontaneous position a child adopts in a hip carry perfectly orients the femoral head into the socket to allow normal development. Recent research suggests that developmental hip dysplasia (DDH) in babies in Malawi who are carried on their mothers' backs in spread-squat positions from 2–24 months is very rare, in contrast to the rate of DDH in infants swaddled into straightened leg positions.[9] Undiagnosed and untreated DDH can cause discrepancies in leg length, a decrease in agility and painful hip and spine arthritis by early adulthood.

As you can see, carrying babies is normal for the human species, and contributes to health and wellbeing. The evolutionary pattern helps to explain why babies naturally expect and want to be carried by their parents. It is part of their biological and evolutionary history. However, carrying a child 'in arms' is hard work for prolonged periods, especially as they grow. Small babies are light enough to be carried in their tucked-up sleepy position in arms on the front, resting against the chest or shoulder and on the parent's forearms, when families are on the move. At this stage in their lives babies are passive passengers, but as they grow heavier frontal in-arms carrying becomes taxing and energy-inefficient. Yet early humans were hunter-gatherers and needed to remain on the move and able to flee from danger. An ape infant who could cling on to his mother was able to travel with her as she moved; a pre-walking human child who could not help his mother by clinging on to her would have become burdensome and possibly a survival risk.

There has been some discussion in recent years about whether early humans used tools to make carrying their offspring easier and less energy intensive. As one paper reported, 'The burden of carrying an infant in one's arms is on average 16% greater than having a tool to support the baby's mass and seems to have the potential to be a greater energetic burden even than lactation.'[10] The researchers also noted that in-arms carrying shortens and quickens the stride of the carrying adult, which also requires greater energy expenditure. 'We suspect that the energetic drain of carrying an infant would be such that some sort of carrying device would have been required soon after the development of bipedalism and definitely to allow long-distance travel, especially that out of Africa and across Asia.'[11]

Anthropologist Timothy Taylor[12] has postulated that the early adoption of carrying aids made from natural materials like animal skins or woven reeds would have eased the burden of this in-arms carrying and allowed further evolution. He suggests that it is both possible and likely that a hominin mother discovered the advantage of some sort of carrying aid by chance. Once a carrying aid had been discovered or invented, early human families with offspring would have been able to move more freely. Such a discovery could have been vital in 'smashing the glass ceiling' in hominin to human evolution. If helpless early human babies, who slowed their families down and sapped their energy, could be quickly and easily carried around, the human race could continue to produce vulnerable babies with larger brains.

Infant humans can be born with as large a cranium as the

maternal upright bipedal pelvis will allow, because their parents and small local societies are able to provide prolonged nurture for many months beyond birth – the 'fourth trimester' of gestation. A sling or carrier acts almost as an external womb, facilitating further maturation until children are coordinated and strong enough to be able to run alongside their families. Brains that are still growing and developing in the outside world are ripe for learning: language, creativity, culture – all the things that make us human. It isn't hard to see how prolonged exterogestation has contributed to the enormous success of the human race.

The world's few remaining hunter-gatherer societies, such as the San Bushmen or some Amazonian tribes such the Awa (who until recently had no contact with the outside world), use slings daily, made from animal skins or woven reeds or cloths; they are simple and allow multiple carrying positions around the wearer's body, as well as feeding. They are a good insight into how our species would have once used slings; to take the child with the parent for easy feeding and allowing prolonged periods of foraging without needing to leave the infant with another carer. Lozoff et al (1979)[13] studied hunter-gatherer societies and found that mothers are the primary caregivers, carrying babies, breastfeeding and providing prolonged bodily contact day and night. They are responsive and nourishing parents, but when not carried children have complete freedom of movement. Despite their intense attachment, the children are quickly independent and by 2–4 years are spending more than half their time away from their mothers. They concluded that carrying is normal behaviour for the human species, and that 'modern' parenting methods of 'caching' (where infants spend little time in contact with their parents, are held in restrictive containers, sleep apart from their families and endure a delayed response to their cries) 'may profoundly alter infant development and maternal involvement'. We ignore our biology at our peril.

The history of modern babywearing

From such simple and intuitive beginnings in early and traditional human societies, the practice of carrying children close to the parent's body has continued, often simply for convenience, rather than to meet children's emotional needs. Indeed, in his book *Parenting for a Peaceful World*, author and psychotherapist Robin Grille surveys the history of childrearing and describes how, for most cultures in history, the wellbeing of children was not the priority it is becoming today.

There are examples of sling use in anthropological and historical records, as well as old photographs. There is evidence that the ancient Egyptians carried babies in slings, and a mediaeval painting, 'The Flight to Egypt' by Giotto (c.1306), depicts the baby Jesus being carried in a sling by his mother Mary.

Simple, easily accessible materials such as plant fibres, animal skins and simple woven cloths have formed the basis of most carrying devices throughout history. These may have great cultural meaning. For example, 'carry nets' in Papua New Guinea, made from pandanus palm fibres, have symbolic roles and are part of womanhood and ancestor rites.

The climate plays a part in choice of carrier. Babies in colder climates may need feeding less frequently due to a reduced requirement for frequent hydration, so can be carried in containers for longer. Communities such as those around the Arctic Circle in Siberia have tended to use 'carry-cots', which are made by families with great care from natural products such as birch bark, in which the limbs of the child can be tightly bound. There are temporary and permanent carry cradles, night cradles and day cradles, all of which have great cultural significance. The Inuit culture use 'amauti' (North American) or 'amaarngut' (Greenland) coats made from seal or caribou skin and fur, with a special pouch inside the coat below the hood where a child can be seated and carried, often all day long. This keeps babies warm in the freezing temperatures. The looseness of the garment means that a travelling mother can easily bring her baby round to the front to facilitate breastfeeding and elimination without exposure to the elements. The Sami people of Norway still use 'komse' carriers: wood and leather cots with hoods and straps that can be carried on the shoulder, or hung from a tree, in which a baby can be safely bound and wrapped in furs (and later, cloths). The carrier is extremely portable and can even be stood on its end, and protects babies from the elements and from harm, being extremely sturdy. Photographs of Native American culture in the late 1800s show children being carried on their mothers' backs inside their clothing, as well as on wooden and leather cradleboards.[14]

In warmer climates mothers tend to use simpler, cooler cloths tied around the body in various ways. Babies may need more frequent feeding for hydration in the heat, so it helps to have them closer to the mother. Cloth weaving is an ancient art used by many cultures around the world. Lengths of woven cloth are multifunctional and serve as clothing, headscarves, sunshades, blankets and labour aids as well as baby carriers. Examples from across the globe include the South American rebozo, the African kitenge and Japanese obi sashes, to name just a few. Although there is little information about carrying in Europe, we do know of traditional Welsh shawls and German Hockmantel garments. These simple lengths of fabric are the ancestors of the wrap-around cloths and ring slings used by Western parents today.

As skills in sewing and cloth decoration have developed, some cultures have created carriers with more formal structures that support a child in a pocket with straps to be tied around the body. These can be beautifully ornate, and some of the best-known examples are Asian, including Chinese mei tai carriers, Korean podaegis and Vietnamese/Thai hmong. For more of the rich history of cultural carrying, consult I.C. Van Hout's book *Beloved Burden: Babywearing Around The World*.

Modern baby carriers in the Western world developed fairly recently; we have simply rediscovered an ancient practice that was lost to us. In the 1960s Ann Moore, a paediatric nurse working for the US Peace Corps, was very influenced by her experience of working in Togo. When she had her first child she attempted to emulate the way the Togoan parents carried their babies on their backs with shawls. However, she found it hard to achieve a secure carry and designed a backpack harness that was the forerunner of the Snugli carrier of 1969, the first 'modern' baby carrier.

In 1971 Erika Hoffman, a mother of four, founded the German company Didymos ('twin' in Ancient Greek). When her infant twin daughters were unsettled she rescued a cloth sling she had brought back from Central America from a cupboard and used it to carry one crying baby. The child calmed and soon the twins loved being wrapped in the cloth as much as Erika enjoyed having them in close contact. She was able to work during the day rather than just in the moments when the twins slept. Other German parents wanted wraps of their own, and Didymos was born; the first woven wrap company and still going strong.

The 1980s saw the development and expansion of the baby carrier market. The first ring sling was made by Rayner Garner, a physiotherapist in Hawaii with an interest in good posture, who wanted to make a more comfortable carrier for his daughter. She had developed heat rash from the artificial fabric of a front pack, but her parents believed strongly in the value of close and loving contact. Unaware of pre-existing slings like the rebozo, they set out to create a flexible and comfortable carrier that allowed the child to adjust her position and posture throughout the day, and enabled discreet breastfeeding, while remaining comfortable for the parent. Their first sling was a woollen scarf that they knotted to form a cross-body pouch, but it needed constant re-tying to be comfortable for both parents. They then folded batik fabric to create an adjustable hammock-shaped carrier threaded through first wooden and then more reliable nylon rings. The ring sling was born.

The practice of 'babywearing' has long been popular among followers of the parenting movement that became known as 'attachment parenting'. This was born from a desire to rediscover a more ancient, natural style of child-rearing. Followers were often not mainstream, and were frequently marginalised or labelled 'hippies'. Today baby carriers are becoming more generally popular, as slings have become more functional and health professionals have begun to stress the importance of close relationships in their conversations with new parents. Companies such as Baby Bjorn have developed effective marketing strategies to bring baby carriers into the public eye and make them more socially acceptable. Many new companies have sprung up in recent years, providing a wide range of comfortable and ergonomic carriers. These have been designed to meet the needs of the baby as well as the carrying parent, incorporating our increasing knowledge of early anatomical development. Alongside the sling manufacturers, a supporting industry of sling and carrier professionals (consultants and libraries) has grown up, born of a strong desire to share rediscovered carrying skills and support new parents.

Despite these innovations and developments, the use of baby carriers is not common in our society, having fallen out of favour a few centuries ago during the rapid social changes of the time. However, attitudes are beginning to change once again.

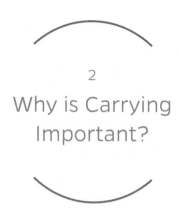

2

Why is Carrying
Important?

'*No species in a hundred years or so can turn the time-tested mother-baby relationship on its head without consequences. In the short term, diminished contact makes babies fussier than they need to be and mothers more conflicted than they need to be. Though the long term consequences are less easily identified, our isolationism, our difficulties with intimacy, our adversarial relationships with our own bodies, all likely relate to a culture that promotes mother-baby disconnection from the beginning and pronounced reduction in close human contact that, even in the most affectionate parent-infant relationships, is still often a mere slice of an infant's day.*'[1]
Sharon Heller, *Vital Touch*

Why does carrying matter? Is it really so important in our modern, fast-paced world where technology provides solutions to every challenge, and engineering ensures everything is as effortless and simple as possible? Our culture prides itself on innovations, space-savers, time-savers, organisation and productivity. There is a whole industry devoted to baby and child products: to keep our little ones secure, to transport them around, to speed up learning and to keep them occupied. The media and our culture encourage us to think that our focus as parents should be on achieving early independence and speedy separation.

In this context, carrying our children and the practice of babywearing matters hugely. In fact, I think it is more important for us now than ever, because of the society we live in and the changes to our culture that have had such an impact on our species. There is a gadget for everything, a pill for every ill; but are we healthier or happier in the long term? Humans are not machines to be managed and controlled and nor are our babies; we are emotional, tactile, social creatures that thrive on contact and communication. In my role as a family doctor I meet many adults who feel broken and abused by the demands of their working and social environments. Time for rest and building relationships is in short supply; yet young babies still need as much love and individual attention as they have always done. Babies long to be carried. They reach for it, they cry for it, and often it is the only thing that brings them peace in the bewildering newness of life. It brings parents peace too.

'I remember the complete bewilderment when my daughter arrived. I can only describe it as clawing to the root of your soul when she clings on to be held. There is something so completely basic and human about carrying.' Emma

Newborn babies respond strongly to touch from their carers. Studies are beginning to show that newborns are genetically predisposed to behave in certain ways to achieve maternal proximity and create contact. Separation from the mother evokes protest, through crying and distressed movements, which is designed to re-establish closeness. Most mothers will respond to crying with an intense urge to soothe their infant's distress by gathering the child into their cradled arms.

Babies appreciate more than just simple touch; movement matters. A recent study has shown that '*infants under 6 months of age carried by a walking mother immediately stopped voluntary movement and crying and exhibited a rapid heart rate decrease, compared with holding by a sitting mother*'.[2] We all know that rocking and swaying an unhappy infant often brings calmness; such movement is instinctive and many of us find ourselves walking up and down in the small hours to help babies fall asleep. Imagine what it must have been like for the baby during the last month or two of pregnancy: dark, warm, contained within soft flexible walls, rhythmic movement, the muffled sound of a heart beating and blood pulsing, regular breathing, the quiet tones of a voice. Birth is a dramatic and overwhelming ejection into space, brightness, noise, sudden stillness and rapid movement. No wonder babies relax and calm when they are placed on a warm chest that sounds and feels familiar, when they are gently rocked and moved, when they are wrapped and given supportive but soft boundaries. No wonder babies love to be picked up and held close for hours on end and find that sleep comes easily when they are cuddled on the chest; it is the place where they feel safe and secure.

Soothing a crying child, however, is about more than just reducing noise and protecting the social grouping against predators for an evolutionary advantage. Babies need nurturing and care, especially in the early stages of their lives. They are particularly vulnerable during the 'fourth trimester' as their bodies and brains adapt to an outside environment. A baby needs his parents to recognise, understand and respond to his every need. He can only express these needs simply. Young babies do not have the perception or cognitive skills to be manipulative; they can only ask for the attention they need with the tools they have, and keep asking until the need is met.

Maslow's hierarchy of needs is useful here.[3] Once a baby's physiological needs have all been provided for (not hungry, thirsty, cold, hot, bored, tired or in pain), he still needs to feel secure and safe, loved and valued. As we have seen, a crying baby will calm and settle when he is held close to a parent's body and rocked and murmured to; his safety, social and esteem needs are met. Studies into the effects of deprivation in institutionalised children show the negative effect that a lack of loving contact and neglect has on a child's brain; growth is stunted and mental health in adulthood can be significantly impaired.[4]

In the 1990s in Romania, ruling dictator Ceausescu's desire to create a Citizen's Army led him to attempt to boost the population, by banning contraception and abortion. This policy led to a huge increase in children who had to go into state orphanages when their impoverished parents couldn't care for them. The children's basic physical needs were met, but they were not loved. They failed to thrive and their brains looked different from those of other children when scanned. Neglected children have smaller brains than children who are loved and well cared for, and the prefrontal cortex (the social part of the brain) is under-developed.[5] Too much exposure to a lot of cortisol (the stress hormone) in the first three years has a lasting impact; it can be toxic to the development of neural connections in these vital years when pathways are being established, and evidence is growing that excessive cortisol in the early years can have many long-lasting negative health impacts, including obesity and heart disease.[6] A child's experiences can alter their thought processes and neural pathways and have a major impact on their future.[7] The good news is that if a child's circumstances change before they are six months old a lot of the early damage can be reversed.

I'm not suggesting that if our children are not carried they will fail to thrive; nor am I suggesting that if children grow up in poverty their emotional development will be stunted. These are extreme cases and the neuroscience is still emerging. Evidence remains sparse and the data needs to be interpreted cautiously. But love and close contact clearly make a difference to children's physiological and emotional development, and with all the innovations and technology available we run the risk of keeping children at arm's length, not giving them our touch, our time and our love – a love that requires our presence and our interaction through close and frequent contact.

Let's look at some of the mechanisms by which close contact and carrying help babies to thrive. Building and developing a loving, trusting relationship of safety and security begins at the moment of birth. A mother will instinctively seek out her newborn infant and hold them close to her heart, just as animals lick their babies all over at birth. This sensory input starts the bonding process.

Physiology

Smell is one of the strongest and earliest senses to develop in a newborn, and the scent of amniotic fluid bears the hallmark of the mother, making her recognisable to a newborn placed on her bare chest immediately after delivery.[8] Warmth and touch also provide essential cues to begin the necessary imprinting (mediated by the release of the hormone oxytocin) to form relationships. The importance of skin-to-skin contact for both mother and baby is well established; UNICEF and the World Health Organisation recommend that all babies remain skin-to-skin for at least the first hour after birth. Babies who enjoy this early skin-to-skin contact experience improved thermoregulation and temperature maintenance, cardio-respiratory stability with apnoea reduction, higher blood glucose levels, facilitated self-attachment for breastfeeding and reduced distress responses to painful stimuli.[9]

In the longer term, infants who had this normal human skin-to-skin contact were found to have shorter lengths of stay in the NICU, fewer infections at six and 12 months, were smiling more often at three months, were ahead of their counterparts in social, linguistic and fine/gross motor indices at one year and displayed earlier urinary continence. Improved brain maturation and better emotional and cognitive regulatory abilities have been noted, as well as more efficient arousal at three and six months (arousal means being awake, alert and able to respond to surroundings). Secure attachments were more likely to have developed between parent and child, and infants were twice as likely to breastfeed compared to those in incubators. Weight gain was greater and sleep deeper.[9,10]

Early skin-to-skin contact is also vital for initiating and maintaining breastfeeding. Babies placed on the mother's bare breast immediately after birth are twice as likely to successfully breastfeed and gain weight better. Breastfeeding is the normal, biological way for a human infant to receive perfectly balanced, responsive nourishment that is kind to their immature gastrointestinal tract. The mother's antibodies (which provide protection from common diseases) are transferred in breastmilk, and breastfed infants enjoy a significantly increased amount of time in skin-to-skin contact, with the subsequent oxytocin release important in bonding and attachment.

A 2012 Cochrane review of studies[11] showed that babies exposed to skin-to-skin contact soon after birth interacted more with their mothers and cried less than babies receiving standard hospital care. Cardiorespiratory stability seemed to be improved. Mothers were more likely to breastfeed in the first one to four months, and tended to breastfeed longer. Babies were possibly more likely to have a good early relationship with their mothers, but this was difficult to measure. Other reviews have begun to show formal evidence of skin-to-skin contact resulting in reduced neonatal mortality.[12]

After decades of research, the ancient practice of holding small or premature babies on the mother's chest, and carrying them carefully inside clothing, especially if they are born small or early, has been adopted by Western medicine and is now known as 'kangaroo mother care'. Many hospital trusts offer this kangaroo care in their special care baby units, and most neonatal units provide opportunities for parents to hold their newborns as soon as possible and for as long as possible before cutting the cord or weighing. The British NICE guidelines for care of the postnatal mother and baby, including after a caesarean section, formally recommend early skin-to-skin and no separation of the woman from her baby within the first hour.[13]

Skin-to-skin even for one hour can be very helpful in reducing maternal stress after birth, particularly when a baby has to spend time in neonatal intensive care. Several recent studies have measured women's stress levels before and after skin-to-skin contact and found a decrease in reported stress as well as reduced salivary cortisol.[14]

Attachment

Harlow's well-known, if unethical, experiments in the 1950s and 1960s into the importance of attachment in rhesus monkeys helped to show that attachment was not dependent on the provision of food (behavioural theory of attachment), but on the provision of soft touch and emotional comfort. Eight infant monkeys were raised with one of two 'mothers' – one made of wire, the other covered in soft cloth. In one setting, the wire mother held food and the cloth mother was empty-handed, while in the other setting the cloth mother had food and the wire mother had nothing. All the monkeys spent most of their time clinging to the cloth mother, even if she had no food. They would only go to the wire mother when they were hungry. If a frightening object was placed near the infant monkeys, they would all retreat to the cloth mother, and the infants were more willing to explore their surroundings when the cloth mother was present. The cloth mother provided a 'safe base' for the infants. These experiments supported the evolutionary theory of attachment; contact and security were most important in creating bonds, rather than the simple provision of food.

These early studies led to Bowlby's conceptual description of attachment and Ainsworth et al's work in the 1970s[15,16,17] watching how toddlers coped with separation from and reunion with their parents in a longitudinal study of mother-infant dyads in the first year of life. It is worth looking at some of Ainsworth's findings in detail.

Mothers who had provided their babies with plenty of affectionate bodily contact during the early months had infants who, by their first birthday, were used to tender and close interaction and were content to be put down, turning 'cheerfully to exploratory behaviour and play activities, demanding relatively little contact under normal circumstances'. These infants were also less likely to protest against their mother's brief absence, showing a tendency to follow her rather than wail in distress.

The researchers contrasted this settled, confident behaviour with that of infants who had experienced relatively little physical contact, especially if this contact was brief, rushed or quickly terminated. These infants tended to protest much more at separation and found it harder to play independently. These children also showed 'great ambivalence about physical contact, sometimes seeking it, but not really enjoying it when getting it'. They were more unwilling to let their mother out of their sight and were often distressed by her departure, suggesting a lack of confident trust.[18]

There is now a wealth of observational evidence and increasing amounts of neurobiological evidence to support the importance of attachment, and hopefully many more clinical studies will follow. We know that human babies who grow up in neglect and deprivation, and are not provided with affectionate parental contact and loving nurture, grow less well (otherwise known as 'failure to thrive'). Disordered or disturbed attachment has been shown to lead to major problems later in life; some studies show that inadequate attachment 'frequently underlies drug and alcohol addiction, homelessness, criminality and mental health problems'.[19]

It seems clear that consistent, appropriate loving touch really does matter in the long term, both at the individual family level and in wider society. Close contact and responsive nurturing does not lead to the clinginess and neediness our society has come to fear, but in fact will guard against it.

'In sum, the presented findings provide support for the assertion that a caring and affectionate approach to infant care that is sensitive to the child's needs and provides physical closeness is more likely to produce secure and ultimately independent children, than a parenting style that overemphasizes independence by limiting physical closeness, at an age when dependency needs are most natural and in fact a sign of healthy psychological development.'[20]

Parents who carry their children frequently are able to provide prolonged periods of close contact, and are often more aware of their child's subtle cues and thus respond more quickly to needs. This 'in-tune' behaviour builds trust and confidence on the part of the child, leading to increased confidence and competence in parenting. It is a mutually beneficial symbiotic relationship. Parents who have a close, physically intimate relationship with their children enjoy the ongoing release of oxytocin, which can help reduce stress and depression and strengthen family bonds. Well-attached children may have a more comfortable personal path through life.

'The single most important child rearing practice to be adopted for the development of emotional and social healthy infants and children is to carry the infant on the body of the caretaker all day long.'[21]

Carrying and close contact are more important even than breastfeeding in promoting physical and emotional health,[22] and whole families flourish when attachment bonds are secure. Being close to you is how your baby will learn about himself and the world he lives in. He will learn to smile in your arms and laugh into your delighted eyes. He will be rocked to sleep in security while hearing a steady heartbeat. He will learn confidence and trust from mutually reciprocated loving touch. He will learn everything important from you. Your tiny child will learn how to engage with the world based on his observations of your reactions to it; he will respond to people his parents have a positive connection with, learning from your welcoming gestures and smiles to people, and be more fearful of those who do not respond (this is known as social referencing or triangulation). He will learn to recognise and manage risk in his daily life, and the strong attachments he forms will be the means to his later independence. He will seek to recreate attachments that seem to have gone awry, based on his positive experience of social interaction.

This is well demonstrated in Tronick's 1975 'still face experiment',[23] in which a mother with a well-attached baby refuses to respond to his cues of play. First he tries to engage her in play, then he tries to encourage her to connect with him, then he bursts into distressed tears when she fails to respond and turns away. He is aware of the lost relationship and feels the coldness of this loss, as such rejection is alien to him.

Ideally we would all carry our babies in our arms, sharing this 'beloved burden' with close-knit family living nearby. Such in-arms carrying encourages breastfeeding on demand – providing both nourishment and nurture, as milk and comfort are easily accessible. In-arms carrying is good for our bodies too, as it keeps us moving and active, using muscles and joints constantly rather than remaining in the same place for prolonged periods. Nourishing movement, good posture and standing well are important for our own health and wellness. We are not sedentary creatures by nature of our evolutionary biology; our bodies need to be upright and in motion for much of the waking day. Carrying a child in arms encourages us to move and change position frequently as we feel their weight pulling at our bodies, and inappropriate postures and overloaded muscles trigger pain signals and keep us shifting the load around. The more we carry, the more our muscles and joints and bones adapt to this regular load and we become stronger. Shifting baby from side to side, from hip to hip, facing in and facing out, on to the back and so on, in an active, fluid motion, all helps to keep the weight distributed, building up our overall strength as the child gradually gains weight. Being in motion around our bodies allows children to be in different positions frequently. This is good for babies; the chance to experience different viewpoints when they are awake and active means they can learn about the world from different positions and exercise different muscles against gravity, giving the vestibular canals a wider range of use.

With all this in mind, it is sobering to see how, in our more recent history, with increasing industrialisation and the devaluing of child-rearing, the frequency and duration of a child's physical contact with his parent has rapidly declined.

Why are so few babies carried?

What is stopping us from carrying our children as much as they need? Exclusive-in-arms carrying is hard to achieve in our society for many reasons. Modern babies spend more time physically separated from their parents than at any other time in history. The maternal body is no longer the primary habitat for human infants, and in-arms carrying is now tiring for our changed bodies. Parents are encouraged to put their babies down and regain their old lives; babies are expected to learn independence as quickly as possible. This approach to caring for children is new in human history and runs counter to attachment theory.

Families in the West are encouraged to remain 'in control' and not to be 'manipulated' by their tiny infants. They are expected to be 'economically active' as soon as possible, and are directed towards achieving uninterrupted periods of sleep, parent-led scheduling and early childcare. Breastfeeding rates have fallen rapidly as close-knit communities, which provide support and encouragement, have fragmented. Cleverly designed advertisements for formula milk subtly undermine breastfeeding and suggest that a return to pre-baby life is the ideal. This has dramatically altered public perceptions of normal baby sleep rhythms and feeding patterns, and encouraged a belief that babies will be spoiled if they are carried everywhere. Post-natal depression is worryingly common, but a continued sense of stigma and failure prevents parents from seeking help. Parents are bombarded with a dizzying array of 'containers': prams, playpens and bouncy chairs. Toys and 'learning tools' distance parents further from their children. Our knowledge of normal baby and parent behaviour is being eroded.

Further, in industrialised societies people are more sedentary than in the past. Poor posture makes us more prone to pain and we take longer to recover from pregnancy and birth, as well as from injury. Carrying heavy loads for prolonged periods is harder than it used to be, and there is thus an increasingly common perception that babies are 'too heavy' to carry.

All this combined means that our babies are carried much less, breastfed much less and experience far less intimate close contact than they need for normal development.

It is interesting to look at some of the data on parent-infant contact in different cultures and across history. For 99 per cent of human existence we lived in hunter-gatherer societies. A few of these nomadic peoples remain, and children are carried and held for more than 50 per cent of their day before the onset of crawling or walking. Mothers and children sleep in the same room – mostly in the same bed – and weaning from the breast comes after the second birthday, often much later. This is an insight into how human beings have lived and cared for their children for millennia. Subsistence cultures (fishing, agriculture, herding) are more recent, and less nomadic, but children are still carried and held a great deal. Nursing and bed-sharing rates also remain very high.

Modern-day post-industrial cultures are very different. The Industrial Revolution transformed attitudes to children and their roles in society. The expectation and demand for increased productivity from adults necessitated earlier independence for children and many natural parenting principles, which are time-consuming, were swept away as communities changed. Village communities and groups of extended family were fractured as people followed the work to the cities; nuclear families became more common, with reduced opportunities for shared childcare and extensive nurture. Many children had to begin working very young, either in industry or in caring for younger siblings, and independence was prized. Soon mothers were encouraged not to pick babies up for fear of spoiling them, and 'excessive' displays of parental affection were frowned upon as unhealthy. *'Nothing is more opposed to true maternal love than the excessive fondness apt to be displayed in caresses, with which, upon all occasions, a mother is tempted to humour the caprices of a little child,'* admonished *Cassell's Household Guide*, published in 1869. Too much physical touch was thought to weaken children and hinder their development.

Beginning in the Victorian era, childbirth began to move out of the home into hospital, prompted by increased knowledge of infection and the rise of medical and surgical specialists. There were good reasons for this; many women died in labour and in the post-partum period, and improved infection control and medical techniques saved many lives. However, the increasing medicalisation of childbirth brought with it a trend towards reduced skin contact and bottle-feeding, while infants were held less and prams and sleeping containers became more popular. Furthermore, popular philosophies at the time meant that breastfeeding began to be regarded as a lower class activity and one that necessitated 'privation and penance' – mothers were thought to be sacrificing cultured social activities and pleasure to nourish their babies. 'Hand-feeding' became much more common in the second half of the 19th century and breastfeeding and 'natural' parenting practices declined.[24] The upper and middle classes began to use nurseries and nannies. *'Children were separated from adults to give them a sheltered and structured routine and to train their character,'* writes Sally Mitchell in *Daily Life in Victorian England*.

Today's infants therefore have a completely different introduction to life than their forebears. Their first habitat is no longer their mother's body. Data from Lozoff and Brittenton[25] shows that traditional societies carried or held their children for more than 50 per cent of their day, but in 1986 a Canadian study demonstrated that babies were carried by their primary caregivers for only 2hrs 40mins a day between three weeks and three months of age.[26] A British study in 2000[27] showed that mothers spent an average of only 61 minutes in 24 hours holding their sleeping or crying child at six weeks of age. This figure was just 17 minutes when the child reached one year old. When feeding contact was added to the data, six-week-old infants spent an average of 3hrs 27mins out of 24 hours in contact with their mothers, and 2hrs 23mins at one year old. The Ainsworth data from 1972[28] suggested that in the first three months of life, close bodily contact with the primary caregiver during waking hours was 35 per cent, and at one year old it had declined to 10 per cent.

These are small studies and need to be interpreted with caution, but it is clear that the normal prolonged and frequent close contact that our infants once enjoyed has dramatically declined.

Socioeconomic factors – making modern life work

Parenting is presented to many in the Western world as a matter of choice. Culture and technology have brought about many changes, and the pressure society exerts on us to be productive and 'successful' creates many tensions.

We live in a society that focuses on success, achievement, personal self-fulfilment and material ownership. There is little respect for those who opt out of such a lifestyle; stay-at-home parents and those who choose or are able to work part-time are often looked down on and envied in equal measure. In my work as a GP I meet many people struggling with the relentless demands of their jobs and the expectations of their peers. There is very little slack in the system to allow for illness, and caring for children is not recognised as a valuable investment in the future.

Our culture has reduced the amount of time people are able to spend in person with each other building relationships and communities that offer support when problems arise. If parents, especially fathers, are expected or need to return to full-time work within a few weeks or months of birth, the opportunities for bonding with the new baby are drastically reduced. If mothers are expected to regain their pre-baby lives and bodies within months of birth, they will make choices to fit into the prevailing culture, rather than choosing to meet the needs of their baby first and foremost. The time that parents have to spend with their children can be significantly reduced, with knock-on psychological effects in later life. This is hardly surprising, as the parent-child bond is the first relationship most of us have, and the most essential of all. Building this bond takes time, which is in short supply. Many parents don't feel they have the time or the support to feed babies whenever they express hunger, to respect their natural sleeping patterns, or to carry children everywhere. They often feel they need to 'restore order' as soon as possible. Thus children are expected to become independent far earlier than is biologically appropriate: weaning from breastfeeding and an end to bed-sharing tends to occur at the age of three to four in traditional cultures.[29]

However technological our world has become, human beings remain organic animals and not machines. It is unsurprising, therefore, that in our pressurised, fractured and isolated society, as the quality of our relationships and connections declines, mental illness is common. Post-natal depression affects at least 10–15 per cent of new mothers, with many more sufferers (and fathers) remaining undiagnosed. Good support can be hard to find, either from families or local communities, or from healthcare professionals. Many affected parents can feel a sense of dissociation and detachment from the child they want to love so much, which can significantly reduce the time they spend carrying or in any close contact.

Changing body shapes and strength

As we have seen, our modern bodies are more sedentary than those of our ancestors. We spend a great deal of time sitting down and resting in poor positions. Our centres of gravity and our mechanical axes are incorrectly aligned, creating strain on joints that were never meant to be weight-bearing at these angles; we move as if we were in a constant 'forwards fall'.[30] Many adults are unaware of how little they move in daily life, compared to our forebears or even active young children, and are rarely mindful of their posture when walking, standing or sitting. Inactive bodies are less flexible; joints are stiffer and more prone to misalignment, which makes carrying weights more uncomfortable. Positively heeled shoes and forward leans tilt the pelvis and create strain on the back, and carrying a weight on the front, hip or back will only increase this loading if it is not done thoughtfully.

Excess body weight is a common cause of back and joint pain and reduced strength. Unfortunately people often find themselves in a vicious circle of pain and reduced mobility and activity, less and less able to carry loads, with an attendant belief that their babies are too heavy or that they just aren't strong enough. This has consequences for mood and motivation.

Women's bodies in our culture are often unprepared for pregnancy, labour and birth, and can take a long time to recover fully (if they do). Carrying a heavy load (a bump or a baby) can be much more of a strain on the spine and abdominal and psoas muscles than it should be. Pelvic floors are often weak and loose, diastasis recti is common, and the exaggerated lumbar lordosis many women adopt (with compensatory thrust-forwards ribs) puts great strain on the non-weight-bearing joints of the body, leading to pain and discomfort later in life.

Loading joints incorrectly makes us weaker and more prone to osteoporosis and fractures; it is easy to see why healthcare and fitness professionals constantly exhort us to move more.

Thus we bear the weight of our babies much less than is normal for the human animal, and we have come to rely on alternative means of providing security and transport, including car seats, prams, bouncy chairs and playpens. These have their advantages, but they also distance parents from their babies as well as reducing opportunities for us to build up our strength and improve our movement. Carrying bulky car seats, with the strain on the spine it produces, or pushing prams with our bodies in a strong forwards lean, both add to our discomfort and further reduce opportunities for physical interaction with our children.

In-arms carrying, in contrast, allows us to shift the baby from one hip to the other, frequently adjusting the load over different parts of our bodies. The discomfort of carrying a load encourages us to move that load somewhere else, allowing tired muscles and joints to rest and gradually building endurance, muscle efficiency and bone strength. Such readjustment of position and location is better for us and our babies than remaining in the same position for prolonged periods, especially as children get heavier.

Babies' bodies experience more movement in a parent's arms or a comfortable sling than in a pushchair or car seat. The natural rhythms of walking and balance, moving limbs against gravity and changing vantage points encourage proprioceptive development and learning.

Reduced breastfeeding rates
Breastfeeding – for nourishment and nurture – is on the decline in modern cultures, despite the fact that it is the biologically normal way for human mothers to feed their babies. Breastmilk

provides a perfectly balanced diet of nutrients, food and fluids, as well as allowing the transfer of antibodies, but for many reasons fewer and fewer babies are breastfed for any length of time.

Breastfeeding is intimately linked to the release of oxytocin, as is skin-to-skin contact, so it is no surprise to find that babies who are carried are much more likely to be breastfed, and for longer, than their non-carried counterparts. Many women find that the intimate closeness of their baby is the trigger for milk let-down, and many babies find that skin-to-skin contact stimulates their desire to feed. Lactation consultants often recommend bare-breasted skin-to-skin contact to establish breastfeeding and help resolve challenges.

The reduction in breastfeeding, and a decreased expectation in families that they will breastfeed when they have a baby, is linked to a reduced likelihood of close contact. Families in hardship and on low incomes are least likely to breastfeed and to carry (though there are many exceptions), and thus miss out on many of the natural bonding mechanisms our bodies create.

Using a sling, especially a soft and mouldable one like a stretchy wrap or a skin-to-skin top, is a good way to encourage frequent and prolonged close contact and thus successful breastfeeding. Some women use their sling as a breastfeeding aid, to reduce the strain on the back from holding a baby with one arm. A sling can facilitate a baby's bond with a father or another trusted caregiver, allowing the mother to have a chance to rest and regain energy for more milk production.

If breastfeeding is impossible or brought to an abrupt and early end, skin to skin and the use of a soft sling will trigger the oxytocin cascade to promote the vital bonding process.

'He was screaming and continually hungry, I was distraught and felt a complete failure because I could not give him the milk he so desperately needed. I placed him

on my bare chest and tucked the duvet around both of us. I felt him relax instantly. He looked up at me with those beautiful, innocent newborn eyes, and complete trust that his needs would be met.' Lizzie

Public perception of carrying and babywearing

Given the current trend for our Western society to prize early infant 'independence' and expect children to fit into our busy lives, anything that seems to counter this culture can be viewed with suspicion and criticism. Everyone has their own ideas about the role children should play in their parents' lives, the amount of time parents should devote to childrearing, and differing values and personal experiences, all of which contribute to a particular, personal perspective.

Parents who carry their children a lot are often warned about 'spoiling' their offspring and creating 'clingy' babies at the expense of the child's emotional security. This is similar to the popular belief that babies need schedules and routines, which mirrors societal pressure on parents to return to their old lives as soon as possible after birth.

Evidence is emerging that children who have formed strong attachments to their caregivers in the first year are much more likely to be confident individuals later in life. A study of 9–11 year olds in an American school showed that 'secure attachment and maternal secure base support were related to higher levels of positive mood, more constructive coping, and better regulation of emotion in the classroom, with effects stronger for emotion regulation than for mood.'[31]

Carrying your child or using a sling will not make your child clingy; it will allow them to develop at an appropriate pace and display normal biological human behaviour, until they are ready to take their first confident forays into the world. Sociocultural influences cause parents to train their children to reduce their need for frequent close interaction sooner than is really normal. (See Chapter 3 for more on this.)

Some believe, as we have seen, that our bodies are not strong enough to carry babies around and, by extension, that parents who choose to carry are somehow 'martyrs' or 'slaves' to their offspring, enduring discomfort to avoid any kind of crying. Nothing could be further from the truth; a good sling makes carrying a pleasure for parent and child, reducing crying and promoting calm enjoyment of each other's company.

Another common belief is that older children who enjoy being carried are 'lazy' and need to be encouraged out of the habit. However, most children who can move independently do not want to be in carriers for prolonged periods. Sometimes children need to be contained for their own safety (crossing the road, for example) or to allow a parent to get to a destination on time. Many toddlers spend a lot of time in pushchairs without similar criticism, and the occasional piggyback for a preschooler also passes without comment; children of all ages will enjoy the close contact with their parents for a short while until they are ready to be off and running again.

The more parents carry their children in public, and the more normal it becomes, the less people will fear creating clinginess or hurting themselves. Over the last five years there has been a significant upturn in the use of slings and carriers, and sling libraries and sling professionals (see page 145) are becoming increasingly common.

Using a carrier does not mark you out as a particular type of parent, who subscribes to particular cultural beliefs; it simply means that you are choosing to keep your child close, according to your biological instinct and their biological needs, making life work in the best way you can.

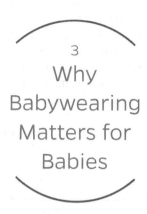

3
Why Babywearing Matters for Babies

Being carried (in arms or in a sling) is normal human behaviour. It is the relationship of closeness and loving touch, as well as the supportive position adopted in confident carrying that matters most, not the type of sling or the fabric. Let us examine in more detail how carrying helps babies to thrive.

The majority of research into the effects of touch and skin-to-skin contact has been done with premature and small babies. Medical studies continue to show that early skin-to-skin and close contact (kangaroo care) improve outcomes for tiny babies. A UNICEF-funded review of 2010 states: *'This evidence is sufficient to recommend the routine use of KMC for all babies under 2kg as soon as they are stable. Up to half a million neonatal deaths due to preterm birth complications could be prevented each year if this intervention were implemented at scale.'*[1]

The World Health Organization (WHO) recommends the frequent use of slings as part of kangaroo care 'for almost every small baby' and illustrates how simple wraparound slings can be used to facilitate skin-to-skin contact between premature babies and their parents.[2] There is no reason why every maternity hospital should not encourage immediate contact between mother and child and more and more NHS trusts are beginning to adopt the principle. One of the 2015 World Health Organization Sustainable Development Goals is to reduce maternal and infant mortality by up to 75 per cent, and kangaroo care will be vital in achieving this target.

The research into kangaroo care has helped us to understand that full-term, healthy babies experience the same positive effects of being carried as their premature counterparts.

Emotional effects

Being carried helps to meets baby's strong need for a sense of security and attachment. Keeping baby close facilitates the parent's speedy response to their needs, thereby building trust.[3] Stressful situations and the frequent, prolonged release of cortisol and adrenaline can be harmful to the developing brain, but this can be countered by prolonged close contact. If parent and child have been separated for any length of time due to medical procedures, incubation, illness or caesarean deliveries, this aid to bonding is particularly valuable. Fostered and adopted children can benefit too; carrying allows the steady creation and consolidation of a new attachment.[4]

> *'The feeling of being completely helpless is still fresh in my mind, I just love though how wrapping them instantly stops the crying and more often than not they will just peacefully fall asleep.'* Katie

Physical effects

Skin-to-skin contact helps to regulate heart and respiratory rates. This is important for children who are unwell, as it results in fewer cases of bradycardia and tachycardia,[5] as well as helping to settle erratic breathing. Close contact is known to enhance growth and weight gain in premature babies and newborns. Cortisol levels remain low when babies are held close, enabling them to conserve energy that can be used for growth and development.[6] Skin-to-skin plays an important role in establishing early breastfeeding, and babies given early close contact are breastfed for longer than their counterparts.[7,8] Skin-to-skin in the first hour after birth, with milk expression, has been shown to significantly increase the volume and speed of milk production for infants with a very low birthweight (compared to those who had a delayed start of 1-6hrs).[9] Breastmilk is babies' normal biological food, and is perfectly adapted to their immature gastro-intestinal systems. It contains valuable disease-fighting antibodies, reduces the incidence of respiratory and ear infections and reduces the risk of diarrhoea (compared to formula-feeding). Breastfed babies seem to be more protected from dental caries, eczema and some childhood cancers, and are less likely to be obese. Therefore, anything that encourages breastfeeding is to be supported.

Babies are unable to regulate their own temperatures effectively. An adult's skin will respond to baby's proximity and alter its own temperature, helping to reduce fever or increase warmth in babies who are skin-to-skin. A parent's naked skin can raise or reduce the infant's temperature by as much as one degree[10] and a parent's skin can respond to the differing temperatures of twins placed on either side of their chest!

Regular close skin contact is believed to help babies regulate their circadian rhythms and distinguish between night and day sleep. We all know that babies sleep well when carried in arms; even more so when motion and noise is involved. Their heart rates slow and breathing stabilises when they are rocked.[11] Babies sleep where they feel safe and secure, and they remain calmer and sleep more deeply and for longer periods when held close.[12,13]

Carried babies seem to cry less. The 1986 Hunziker and Barr study[14] suggested that extra carrying, initiated prior to an expected peak of crying at six weeks, eliminated the peak and reduced the amount of crying significantly and steadily from three weeks of age. However, this data was not replicated in two further studies with similar trial designs. Studies into carrying and colic do not show a significant difference in the frequency of episodes of inconsolable crying and colic between babies who are carried and those who aren't. However, a comparative study[15] of London parents (reduced time in close contact, slower to respond to cries, more likely to feed according to schedule), Copenhagen parents (providing more interaction and responsiveness) and parents offering 'Proximal Care' (prolonged close contact, quick to respond to crying and feeding on demand) showed that the London babies fussed and cried 50 per cent more than the Copenhagen or Proximal Care babies, who just fussed rather than cried. Presumably this is because they trusted that their needs would be met without the need for loud crying. Parents who are close to their children pick up on irritable cues before they become full-blown howls; crying is the last stage of communication. Less crying may enhance the parent-child dyad's mutual bonding and understanding of each other, and gives more time for 'quiet absorption', a state that promotes learning and positive interactions with the world.

Such is the power of close contact that babies are able to handle painful procedures with less distress and cry less in response to such stimuli.[16] (Take your baby for his vaccinations in a sling!) Babies with excessive wind can be hard to soothe, but the motion of being gently rocked in arms or a sling often helps to bring up air or to settle an unhappy child.

The symptoms of gastro-oesophageal reflux are often eased by upright positioning, and there may be a reduced risk of ear infections as a result.[17] Affected babies may prefer to sleep upright, and a sling can make it much easier for a parent to meet this need. Furthermore, the spread-squat position of knees above the bottom helps to relax the puborectalis muscle, which aids bowel elimination. We in the Western world have higher rates of bowel dysfunction compared to those who squat for toileting; studies are examining why this is.

The motion experienced by a baby in a sling allows the vestibular balance apparatus to develop more rapidly than in babies who are often motionless in a seat or on the floor. Being moved around enhances a baby's opportunity for motor development and builds their muscle strength. It improves neck and head control, but is not a substitute for 'tummy-time' (when head-lifting is against gravity).

Close skin contact encourages the development of maternal antibodies to pathogens on baby's skin, which are then passed on through the milk, helping to protect baby from these microbes.[18] Ensuring a low level of cortisol in the blood (by frequent touch and reduced stress) may enhance immune function.

Carrying in the natural physiological spread-squat position, and correctly designed slings that encourage this, can help prevent hip problems in children at risk of hip dysplasia. This is discussed in more detail in Chapter 6. Babies who are carried are also at reduced risk of plagiocephaly (the flattening of the skull bones at the back of the head from prolonged periods lying on the back, more common since the 'Back to Sleep' campaign).[19]

Social effects

There is evidence that babies' interaction with their caregivers is enhanced by close contact and that their communication and speech benefit. Focal length (how far away a baby can focus his or her eyes) is short for the first few weeks of life and at six weeks is no further than the distance from breast to face. Being held in close proximity gives baby the chance to begin focusing on faces and hearing encouraging speech sounds, which stimulates the desire to mimic and see the positive reinforcement of such attempts. Carrying is thought to encourage sociability; being able to hear the parent's voice and watch their interactions with the world and other people is beneficial and helps cement family relationships.

Being carried allows the baby to retreat from an overwhelming world and snuggle into the parent's body for respite, peeping out from a safe place in a way that isn't possible if they are lying on the floor or in a seat.

A study in Nova Scotia[20] randomised 100 mothers and their full-term healthy babies to two groups. One was given no instructions about baby care, and the other was asked to provide skin-to-skin contact with their naked infants (apart from a nappy) on their bare chests as much as possible. The second group maintained contact for five hours a day in the first week and three hours a day for the next three weeks, whereas the first group provided little or no skin-to-skin contact. The babies were studied at one and three months, assessing the quality of their attachments and how they behaved in the 'still face' experiment (see Chapter 2).

One-month-old babies in the control group did not really engage with the 'still face' experiment, as they had not yet developed expectations of parental behaviour. However, the babies exposed to prolonged skin-to-skin contact exhibited distress at their mother's unresponsiveness (as you would expect to see at three months). At three months, the control group was beginning to show signs of distress during the still phase, as expected, but the skin-to-skin babies actively attempted to re-engage the mother, which would not normally be expected until nine months. The researchers suggested that skin-to-skin in the early months had allowed these very young babies to learn, earlier than previously believed possible, how to regulate their stress and request attention or change by reacting positively with vocalisations to engage the parent rather than crying in distress. Further studies continue to bear this out, showing that prolonged close contact in the early months of life gives babies an advantage in neurological development.

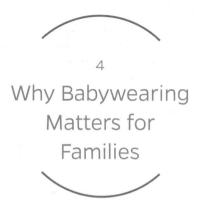

4

Why Babywearing Matters for Families

Carrying and close contact are important for parents and caregivers too and play an important part in emotional and physical health, as well as being convenient and giving parents their hands back to get on with daily life.

Attachment for the mother

It is not just babies who need to form relationships; parents need to feel intimately attached to their offspring to be able to invest their time and energy. Again, it is oxytocin that plays a major role in creating this emotional connection, via many pathways. This is one reason why babies should be placed on their mothers' bare chests immediately after delivery: skin-to-skin, and the scent of the baby, helps the parent to bond. This can be especially important after caesarean sections, or long and difficult labours, where the natural cascades of oxytocin and prolactin during labour and birth may have been attenuated. Prolonged separation from tiny premature babies can also make bonding difficult, and every effort should be made to enable parents to hold their babies. The NICE guidelines[1] on the care of the mother after a caesarean say that: '*Early skin-to-skin contact between the woman and her baby should be encouraged and facilitated because it improves maternal perceptions of the infant, mothering skills, maternal behaviour and breastfeeding outcomes, and reduces infant crying.*'

> '*Rosie was premature, and the hospital encouraged us to do as much skin to skin as possible. It was a very anxious time for us, but having her little bare self on my bare self was about the greatest thing ever. She slept, and while her heartbeat evened out and her breathing regulated, I relaxed and breathed in her precious baby smell and kissed her little wrinkled head. I remember one such time in the wee small hours of the morning, whispering to her all of the promises I made, about how I would keep her safe and how I would love her and what wonderful things we would do together. That skin on skin was magical, there's really nothing like it. I remember crying one night and being physically unable to move her away from me. It was so hard to have to put her back. I started wrapping when she was about six weeks old and it was like the magic was renewed. She was mine again, and the hours I wore her to help relieve her reflux and calm myself are without number.*' Jodie

In real life not all new mothers and babies are instantly enchanted with each other. Nurturing a newborn can be hard work. There are new skills to master, insistent needs to meet and sleep may be in short supply. Many parents feel anxious about their ability to cope, especially if they have other areas of life where they need to keep on top of things.

A close bond takes time to build, and fortunately oxytocin

release isn't a matter of willpower, but simple chemistry. Hormones are a powerful part of our emotional experience and their release can be triggered by certain behaviours. Holding a baby close, even if you feel detached, will still encourage oxytocin release and begin to build emotions that may feel lacking – baby will feel it too and relax and fall asleep. It is *good* to hold your sleeping baby – as much for your own benefit as for theirs. Don't rush to put them down so you can 'get on with things'. By holding them you are doing an important job: life is ultimately about relationships, and investment in your future mental health and that of your baby is well worth it. Time really does fly – the days may feel painfully long, but the years are short.

> *'Carrying my child is perfect for us both. He has had a tough start in life and could quite easily not have made it. He has a few health problems but I know by carrying him, where he can lay his head on my heart, he feels safe and loved. The closeness we share is the greatest feeling in the world, he's with me and I'm with him and we are content.'* Zara

Frequent close contact helps to build parental confidence. A heightened awareness of baby's little movements and noises and subtle changes in mood will soon help a parent to feel in tune with their child, increasing their responsiveness. Thus the baby learns that her parent is willing to work out what is going on and give her what she needs when she asks, before she cries. There is no reason to delay in meeting a baby's needs: babies are not able to manipulate their parents. They are simply aware of a need, and will call for it to be met, entirely appropriately for their developmental stage. Babies whose needs are met promptly can relax and be calm, which will encourage sleep. This positive feedback cycle is affirming for a parent – a successful response to a child's needs builds confidence and assures them that they are coping well.

> '*Babywearing has always helped me to feel that both Reu and I are safe and secure. When Reu is in the sling, I can easily see that he's safe and all his needs are being met (especially in those early newborn days when everything is new and there's a lot of new things to process and learn about, this was a major reassurance for me). I also feel much happier about my own safety and well-being when Reu is in a sling on me, it feels like we are within our own bubble of safety and comfort together.*' Sally

Attachment in the wider family

Both parents need to bond with their child, not just the mother; both parents need to feel the connection that makes the investment of parenting worth it. Therefore, encouraging fathers and partners to hold and carry their children will build this relationship and make them more likely to be supportive and share the parenting load.

A baby who has bonded with more than one caregiver will be more likely to accept comfort and care from them, rather than exclusively seeking the mother. It is useful to be able to share the care of a baby to ensure everyone is getting the rest and nurture they need to be the best parents they can. Close contact with a child helps to strengthen wider family connections and helps the baby to recognise more people by their voices, appearance and scent, and be more willing to be cared for by others outside the nuclear family.

> '*One of my favourite things about carrying has to be the confidence it has given my partner in his abilities and*

how much it has strengthened their bond.' Alicia

Carrying can be useful when parenting older children who are adapting to changes in their world; they can return to their secure places (close to their parents) for comfort and reassurance. It is valuable for parents to be able to provide stability during transitions and adjusting to new circumstances such as a nursery.

> *'It's those difficult moments that you can make easier by carrying them. My little boy loved the nursery but was exhausted and it was lovely to feel him unwind and recharge on our walk afterwards.'* Cat

Carrying can help to support older siblings as families grow. A baby in a sling means that parents can have their hands free to interact with older children so that they don't feel pushed aside. In fact, many older children want to be in close contact and even to be carried again when a baby is in the house, as a reminder that they are just as loved as they ever were. Being held close to a parent provides some much-needed reconnection and reinforces existing bonds.

> *'Carrying has lessened the upheaval of a little brother arriving into the family on my little girl. We haven't had to stop doing anything or going anywhere because we have a baby. He's included even when he's asleep which I really love!'* Fiona

> *'Carrying our new little boy has meant I can keep him close and still devote time, love and attention to his big sister – as a child of preschool age, she still needs a lot of support, even whilst we cope with the demands of a new baby. Babywearing means less of a need to compromise*

the attention I give to either child, which makes for a happier family all round.' Anna

Close carrying can be a useful tool for adoptive and foster parents. Children in these circumstances may be traumatised and lacking in attachment and rebuilding this can take time. Fortunately, much of the damage done can be corrected by providing stable, reliable and loving relationships. A study by Bick and Dozier[2] tested the oxytocin levels in mothers' urine as they interacted with first their own children and then with unrelated and unfamiliar children (a stressful situation). The results showed that oxytocin levels in mothers were raised during their time with the unfamiliar children, more so than during interactions with their own children. The significance of this difference isn't yet clear, but adds to the growing body of evidence that maternal behaviour is very much hormone-mediated. Oxytocin is produced in response to stress and helps to reduce it; it aids memory and recognition of faces, and it is also known to encourage positive social behaviour and increase empathy and trust towards strangers. Using a sling to carry an unfamiliar child is therefore likely to promote bonding, trust and acceptance, and the child will benefit from the contact and needs-meeting behaviour.

Babywearing and post-natal mood disorders

One of the most important positive outcomes of carrying, for a parent and the society we live in, is the effect it can have on mental health. Mental wellbeing is an underfunded but vitally important area of health. The continued demands that our culture makes on us to be useful and productive, and the way it rewards intense workloads, is, in my view, breaking us as human beings. I see many people in my consulting room who are cracking under the strain of employer expectation, financial constraints, loneliness and the feeling of being unsupported and unvalued. Western society is increasingly fractured and isolated, with a decreased sense of local community and shared care. The burden of mental illness in our society is growing, and becoming a parent in this environment can be very tough indeed. Parents often have to return to work very quickly as maternity pay is inadequate and fathers may get very little paternity leave at all, leaving a mother on her own early in her parenting journey, with little family support.

It is no wonder that post-natal depression is so prevalent, affecting at least 10–15 per cent of new mothers, and probably many more. A surprisingly high number of parents struggle to feel connected with their newborns.

'It is just so hard to face another day of feeling totally unlike myself, missing my old life, unable to enjoy this new one.' Pam

'The worst part was the guilt I felt about crying every day when I had a beautiful new daughter.' Lydia

Parents often feel ashamed to admit their feelings, and the effects of hiding their struggle can have knock-on effects on the whole family.

'My husband felt helpless because he knew something was wrong but I wouldn't admit it and shut him out. All he could do was try to look after me and be there when I finally admitted it. It caused a lot of irrational arguments.' Miriam

Fathers can suffer too.

> *'The first few weeks were the hardest and I would just sit and cry. I felt like this shouldn't happen to me, I should just be taking it on the chin and getting on with it. But the truth is, I felt alone and without the support of my wife, I would've been a lot worse.'* Tim

Babies who cry inconsolably and never seem to sleep can be very distressing for a family and research shows they are more likely to suffer harm from parents at the end of their tether. This is a terrible indictment of our culture and its lack of care for some of the most vulnerable individuals in our communities.

> *'PND is the scariest and loneliest place on the planet and puts a terrible strain on the whole family.'* Rob

Post-natal anxiety is also very common. The fear of not being good enough, or being unable to cope with the enormous change in life a baby brings, can be exhausting.

> *'It isn't about not loving your baby but about feeling overwhelmed with responsibility and unable to cope.'* Al

It is clear that something needs to be done. The way we live now isn't going to change overnight; funding for parental leave and greater support for mental health won't suddenly become available, and the media will continue to bombard us with 'advice' and advertisements for products intended to make the job of parenting easier but that distance us from our children. Nor are the emotional needs of young children going to diminish, especially if we want them to grow up well and happy, to be confident mature individuals who are well integrated into society. We should be encouraging and protecting parents' precious time with their small children; giving children a secure and confident start in life pays dividends later for the whole of society. Luckily we have tools that we can use even when times are tough for parents, and carrying is one of them.

> 'For me the act of tying my child to me calms both of us and is a wonderful diffuser. After twenty minutes of whining, we sat on a bench and I said 'What's wrong?'. He said 'I don't know' then 'Can I have a carry?' He was only up for five minutes but it was all that was needed. He buried his head in the back of my neck and chattered away and all was calm. I know exactly what he means too... sometimes I don't know what's wrong, but I'd love a cuddle myself.'
> Sarah

Recent research has begun to study carrying behaviours and depression. Uvnäs-Moberg (1996) noted that the anti-stress effects of oxytocin are particularly strong when it is released in response to a 'low intensity' stimulation of the skin, i.e. simple touch, which babies can provide to their mothers by simply resting against them. Anisfield et al (1990) noted a lower incidence of post-natal depression in carrying mothers. A study in 2012 (Bigelow) tested the salivary cortisol levels (raised in stress) and two depression scores of mothers who were asked to provide six hours of skin-to-skin to their newborns in the first week and then two hours a day for the next three weeks, with the control group being given no specific instructions about the care of their infants. Salivary cortisol was reduced and the depression questionnaire scores were lower in the skin-to-skin group. The researchers concluded that increased skin-to-skin with their newborns benefits mothers by reducing their depressive symptoms and alleviating physiological stress in the post-natal period.

There is now a steadily growing body of anecdotal

evidence that carrying can be a useful tool for helping parents who are dealing with depression. It is hard to find the motivation to make the effort to interact with a baby who just cries; but the physical act of providing skin-to-skin and carrying (in arms or a sling) can be very helpful medicine for a struggling mother.

'*When she was in her pram I felt completely removed from her and her world. I was just an accessory, she was a job to do and I was irrelevant. Using a sling finally helped me bond properly with her and made a massive difference to the PND.*' Nina

Knowing that a baby often relaxes into a carry gives a tired and worried parent another skill in their parenting toolbox when they feel helpless, and can rebuild their self-belief.

'*There were moments when nothing else but carrying and wrapping would soothe my little girl and she instantly relaxed into me – these moments made me feel like maybe I do know what I'm doing and maybe it will be ok.*' Kathy

Feeling trapped inside the house or unable to participate in enjoyable social activities due to constant feeding makes mothers feel lonely and isolated. Having a carrier in which a baby will settle and maybe sleep gives parents more freedom. It can allow opportunities to do things that need to be done, reducing feelings of falling behind with daily life, or allow them to get out for a walk. Exercise releases endorphins, which contribute to feelings of wellness and can help with weight loss, often an important part of self-esteem. Babies can often be fed in a sling (from the breast or with a bottle), which gives parents choice about how to spend their days, rather than being limited by routines.

'The sling brought us back to an almost pregnant-like state, with him a part of me, listening to one another's cues. He was calmer for being close to me, which made me feel more confident, which brightened my mood. Leaving the house felt less daunting so I got more exercise and again increased my confidence. I talked to him more, whether he was awake or not, and he became my son rather than a tiny scary stranger.' Joni

A baby who hates the car can be carried in a sling on public transport to ensure life doesn't become too limited, reducing the risk of social exclusion. Crowds can become easier to navigate without a large pushchair, which can help with feelings of being in the way or burdensome. Older children can have their needs met more quickly, avoiding tantrums that can add to a parent's feelings of being overwhelmed. Slings can help babies to sleep better and cry less, which can be lifesaving.

'I had post-natal depression with my eldest. She would never sleep in the day and would feed every hour and wouldn't be put down. I didn't know about slings other than high-street carriers which didn't really work well for us. Although I have always loved her fiercely, I found bonding hard. I was simply exhausted and not coping. All the usual denial of PND by myself and family meant it was 10 months before I sought help. It really took over the next few years of my life. I had to 'work' at being the parent I wanted to be. I got my nerve up to try for a second after four years. I came across slings primarily as a practical solution to living in a hilly city and having to do school runs. However, I fell in love with wearing my new baby in a sling. I felt calm with her next to me. She and I would relax into each other. She

slept in the day in the sling, this helped my milk production, she fed well, we co-slept safely – it felt like I was cuddling my baby all the time, giving her what she and I needed. I felt calm and relaxed. I felt motherly and nurturing. My calmness meant that my relationship with my eldest daughter became less tense. My regret was that it hadn't been like this with her, but I now sometimes sleep with her in her bed for the night and we cuddle each other and tell each other how much we love each other. I'm convinced that not being stressed with a baby who wouldn't sleep in the day made all the difference. I have found carrying my second child to be very healing.' Caroline

Physical health

The hormones released when women carry their babies improve their health, promoting uterine involution (the process whereby the uterus shrinks back to its pre-pregnancy size) and reducing the risk of post-partum haemorrhage. As carrying mothers tend to breastfeed exclusively, they may enjoy several months of amenorrhoea (no periods), which helps to preserve iron stores. There can be better blood sugar control and weight loss while breastfeeding, as well as a lower risk of osteoporosis and breast, uterine, endometrial and ovarian cancer.

Back and pelvic pain is common in our society and muscles are often not toned enough for regular load-bearing (although they will adapt with time). A good comfortable baby carrier will spread the weight of a child evenly around the body, supporting your baby in a safe, comfortable seated position while getting on with daily life; being on the move is conducive to good health, both now and in the future.

There is very little information about the effects of infant carrying on the biomechanics of human posture and walking, but more work has been done on the effects of carrying rucksacks, for example. Carrying heavy loads is very taxing on the body and can have effects on the gait of the person carrying. One study[3] demonstrated that a front-carrying parent may try to compensate for the displacement of the centre of mass by taking a larger step forward and not extending their leg fully behind, while carrying in arms, without the use of tools, causes backwards leaning while walking. Back-carrying parents may try to maintain their balance by leaning forward to stabilise the load on their back. Such shifts in load bearing, especially if maintained for a few hours, will be tiring, and in-arms infant carrying is also energetically very expensive. A good comfortable sling, properly positioned, can help to balance weight well and prolong the amount of time a parent can carry before fatigue begins to set in.

The ability to carry a child securely for longer periods of time gives parents more opportunities for physical exercise; many people find that carrying their children on walks helps them to lose weight and tone muscles; and being out in the fresh air is good for the soul and can help to calm a fractious child, contributing to overall family wellbeing. The sling means the pram can be left behind for explorations off the beaten track, or for easier navigation of crowded situations such as shops, public transport and busy airports.

'Carrying matters to me – for creating the most precious bond with our children, for enabling us to get out and about as a family and for the hands-free cuddles that mean I can cook tea, help with homework or play football with the older boy so that family life feels stress-free and filled with love, I love carrying my babies!' Elinor

Of course, it is wise to build up strength gradually after birth to encourage full recovery before taking on the carrying of heavy loads. Ligaments may take a while to firm up after stretching and many mothers' bodies may not be ready for vigorous exercise for a few months after birth. Any kind of prolonged carrying activity should always be undertaken with caution and gentleness. I usually advise parents new to sling use to gradually build up the time they spend using their carrier, allowing their muscles to tone and bodies to adjust to the exercise, just as if they were training for a long race.

> *'We love knowing that we can just go out anywhere, and take our children with us; we aren't limited to flat paths or gentle inclines. We can climb hills up to the top of the world together and enjoy the views across the valleys.'* Rosie

Enjoyment

Carrying children can be great fun and enhance parents' enjoyment of this all-too-brief stage in their lives. Learning techniques for carrying is a chance to acquire new skills and many families find a new social circle within their local sling meets, sharing their love of carrying and learning new things together, in the same way that village societies used to care for each other. Slings can also be beautiful, many can be customised for personal choice, and colour therapy can provide a lift on a difficult day. There are very few hobbies that can benefit a parent so much while bringing so many good things to a baby.

> *'Babywearing has given me a more confident social voice – it's introduced me to an online (and real life) circle of like-minded friends who I feel confident chatting to.'* Harriet

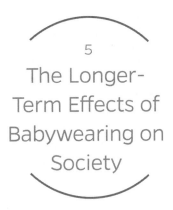

5

The Longer-Term Effects of Babywearing on Society

The effects of improved breastfeeding

There are other benefits to our society when babies are carried. More carrying means more breastfeeding, as breastfeeding rates and duration are higher in carried babies. More breastfeeding means less ill-health for babies and their mothers, and a reduction in strain on the NHS. A 2009 review summarised this:

> '*For infants, not being breastfed is associated with an increased incidence of infectious morbidity, including otitis media [inner ear infection], gastroenteritis, and pneumonia, as well as elevated risks of childhood obesity, type 1 and type 2 diabetes, leukaemia, and sudden infant death syndrome. For mothers, failure to breastfeed is associated with an increased incidence of premenopausal breast cancer, ovarian cancer, retained gestational weight gain, type 2 diabetes, myocardial infarction, and the metabolic syndrome.*'[1]

The WHO Global Strategy for Infant and Young Child Feeding

states that: *'Infants should be exclusively breastfed for the first six months of life to achieve optimal growth, development and health. Thereafter, to meet their evolving nutritional requirements, infants should receive nutritionally adequate and safe complementary foods while breastfeeding continues for up to two years of age or beyond. Exclusive breastfeeding from birth is possible except for a few medical conditions, and unrestricted exclusive breastfeeding results in ample milk production.'*

Feeding a child breastmilk is normal human behaviour; it is not a 'bonus' in the way that a vitamin supplement may be helpful but is not essential. Carrying and close contact are the same; it is not an ideal beyond the norm, it is basic parenting. If skin-to-skin contact and carrying improve breastfeeding rates (as well as improving bonding and reducing post-natal depression), they should be encouraged for every parent.

It is interesting to note that research has shown that mothers who wanted to breastfeed but didn't are at an increased risk of developing post-natal depression, as are low-income mothers, those in minority groups, those with premature or sick babies and those who are already highly anxious. However, these groups are also the least likely to breastfeed or carry their babies, and miss out on the beneficial effects of these practices. This is something that needs to be addressed at a wider socio-political level. Educating those who work with pregnant women and disadvantaged families to encourage carrying (as well as breastfeeding) would benefit whole families and the wider society.

The effects of improved attachment

A sobering review of international attachment studies done by the Sutton Trust[2] (a think tank that aims to improve social mobility through education) found that children under three years old who do not form strong bonds with a parent 'are more likely to suffer from aggression, defiance and hyperactivity when they get older'. They found that up to 40 per cent of children lacked this secure bond with their parents, which was likely to lead to their own children suffering from insecure attachment; a vicious, repeating cycle: '*Parents who are insecurely attached themselves, are living in poverty or with poor mental health, find it hardest to provide sensitive parenting and bond with their babies.*' The review also found that children with weak attachment were more likely to be obese later in childhood (with subsequent effects on their adult health).

There is growing evidence that our society's tendency to be 'adult-led' and less responsive to babies' needs has a negative impact on their later mental health. However, meeting children's needs and allowing them free play helps to develop conscience, empathy and socialisation, improving stress management, reducing aggression and improving resilience. Some paediatric psychologists have begun to postulate that the social practices and cultural beliefs of modern life are actually detrimental to children's healthy brain and emotional development.[3]

It is clear that babies who have been given plenty of close contact and have been parented in a responsive way in their early years are more likely to grow up with strong self-esteem and to enjoy healthy relationships. They are likely to have fewer attachment disorders and less need of child and adolescent mental health services. They may have had fewer ear infections, less corrective treatment for plagiocephaly and have been less of a cost to the NHS budget. As adults they may be more stable and healthy overall, with consequent benefits to society.

Therefore it seems paramount to improve education for healthcare workers involved with parents, especially those in disadvantaged situations. Efforts need to be made to improve attachment relationships and provide parenting tools (for example by encouraging carrying behaviours), thereby improving the future of children who will be tomorrow's adults.

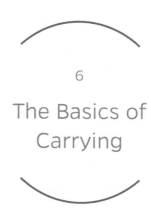

6

The Basics of Carrying

Carrying children safely in soft carriers can be one of the most precious experiences we ever have as parents or caregivers. There is something very special about the closeness that comes from babywearing. But however fantastic it may be, it must be done safely, for your baby's health and your own. Being armed with the knowledge to do this is empowering and builds parents' confidence.

Sling use for very young babies (from birth to four months) is becoming more common in the developed world, echoing the traditional practice of baby carrying around the globe. Families that live in traditional extended communities or 'villages' are usually able to share well-honed, tried and tested knowledge down the generations and provide easily accessible advice and support to new parents. This kind of local support is much harder to come by in our more fragmented modern societies, which means we often turn to books or the internet to fill the gaps in our knowledge and provide us with reassurance we are doing it right. Unfortunately, sometimes these sources of information are out of date or incorrect. Manufacturer instructions can be slow to be updated with new guidelines, and YouTube videos may be misleading or leave out important information. Currently, trained sling consultants and librarians are the most reliable sources of experienced advice and support: they have learned these skills and are keen to pass them on. This chapter gives an overview of the background information and safety considerations that it's helpful to be aware of if you're new to the idea of babywearing.

It's all about the airway

Babies, when they are first born, have not yet begun to develop the secondary curves that will eventually allow them to hold their disproportionately heavy heads up. While they cannot hold their heads up unaided, they need to be supported safely. These early months are the most important in terms of optimum positioning and safety when carrying. It takes time for the spine to change shape so that the baby can sit unaided and walk upright.

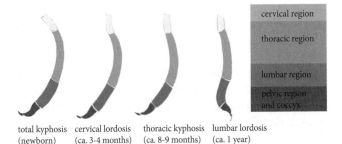

total kyphosis (newborn)   cervical lordosis (ca. 3-4 months)   thoracic kyphosis (ca. 8-9 months)   lumbar lordosis (ca. 1 year)

cervical region

thoracic region

lumbar region

pelvic region and coccyx

The combination of curved spine and heavy head can, if allowed, lend itself to some chest compression and potentially to significant airway compromise; we have all seen babies slumped over in chairs and car seats. Some studies have shown that de-oxygenation can occur in such situations.[1] Chronic or intermittent hypoxia can have negative effects on future development, behaviour and academic achievement, so good position is important.[2] All babies should have their heads well supported and their chins off the chest for optimal breathing. This can be achieved with the instinctive in-arms carrying position, with baby's chest held flush against the parent. The chest support prevents collapse, which also helps to keeps the back supported, and the chin is held off the chest. This looks like a gently curved 'J' shape from the side (as opposed to a 'C' shape).

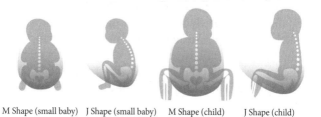

M Shape (small baby)   J Shape (small baby)   M Shape (child)   J Shape (child)

This is why the babywearing terms 'close enough to kiss' and 'visible and kissable' are useful; it's all about airway safety. A parent should be able see their child's face and feel their breathing, allowing them to notice and respond quickly to any changes. A small study by Stening et al[3] showed that there was a very minor decrease in oxygen saturations in those babies who were carried safely in slings compared to those who were laid flat in beds. They concluded that this was 'not associated with an increased risk of clinically relevant cardiorespiratory changes in term and preterm infants.' More clinical studies to assess different positions and their effects would be very valuable.

However, it is clear that babies held low down are at

greater risk of slumping and suffocating. This is why some 'bag-sling'-style carriers have been removed from sale, after deaths due to airway compromise. The shaping of such crescent slings forces the infant to lie curled up inside the sling, with his heavy head pressed forwards onto his collapsed chest or pushed into the parent's breast, rather than seated upright. The fabric over the face reduces airflow and carbon dioxide levels can rise.

Good ergonomic slings keep young babies snug, upright and visible, with fabric away from the face and the back well supported with the chin off the chest. These are the primary tenets of sling safety.

Baby handling

All babies are born with a host of primitive reflexes. As they grow they lose most of them, enabling them to develop greater control over their bodies and integrate all they are learning about proprioception (the knowledge of where their limbs are in space). Carrying a baby respectfully allows the reflexes to diminish and encourages immature vestibular balance organs to develop, allowing a baby's limbs to stretch out in different directions and build up strength. The end result should be a child who has successfully integrated all these involuntary gestures into graceful, co-ordinated movements, with good posture and alignment of the head and spine and limbs; carrying with care promotes good development. A baby who is moved suddenly and perceives a sudden loss of support or a marked change in sensory stimuli will demonstrate the 'Moro' reflex, a rhythmic spreading wide of the limbs followed by a clasping action.[4] The baby will often be startled and begin to cry, due to the feeling of falling.

Reflexes such as the Tonic Labyrinthine Reflex (TLR) and the Landau reflex have a role in helping a newborn to master head and neck and limb control. The TLR can be elicited if a newborn's neck is extended backwards; the baby will automatically stiffen and extend the back further, arching with straightened legs. Holding an older baby (three months plus) in the air, prone around his middle, will trigger extension of the body with head back and legs raised into a backward curl (the Landau reflex). Pressing his head downwards into flexion will make the outstretched legs relax downwards, so baby is curled inwards (one reason why 'bag' slings, where fabric covers the back of a baby's head, can be a suffocation risk). Therefore, handling a child carefully when picking him up, supporting his bottom rather than lifting just around his ribs, and holding him in his naturally adopted positions will help to avoid triggering these reflexes. This will ensure that the baby's movements are active, voluntary and contribute to growth and development, rather than involuntary and jerky. Good handling skills help with confident in-arms carrying and sling use, avoid stressing the infant and build trust.

As babies grow, their neck muscles get stronger and they begin to hold their own heads against gravity. Until then, it is good to respect their natural curved anatomy and avoid straightening spines out too soon. Some harness-style narrow-based carriers on the market put very young babies in straightened positions with arched-back spines and unsupported legs. This is very different to how babies are carried in arms against the parent's chest or in ergonomic slings. These carriers therefore need large and sturdy headrests to support babies who end up leaning back, which is thought to be in part due to their primitive reflexes being activated, and in part because their spines are no longer curled in.

Much of the rigidity or hyperextension seen in some babies in the early weeks and months may be due to pain or distress, such as birth trauma, sore tummy, stiff muscles or an unmet need. This can be really hard for parents to deal with, and such babies and their parents may need time and professional support to be able to relax and settle into more comfortable, confident handling. If your baby seems to be uncomfortable, do seek help from your healthcare professionals. However, if baby is well and healthy and still seems rigid or straight, it may be worth considering whether the posture is due to their reflexes and if a change of handling would help.

Of course, there are always some babies who don't seem to be happy being carried; they may have had difficult births, or be uncomfortable in certain positions due to abdominal pain or muscle issues. A baby should never be forced into a position he does not wish to adopt and it may be wise to seek advice about your baby's choice of positioning.

Sitting comfortably

When you pick up a contented or sleeping newborn, you will see them actively tuck their legs up into a squatting position ready to be carried. They often sleep like this, rest in car seats and chairs in this fashion, and curl their legs up for nappy changes, keeping their spine gently curved and hips slightly apart with knees above bottom, in an 'M' shape. This is biologically normal, a remnant of our evolutionary history, and aids carrying in-arms and on the hip. It is more comfortable to rest on a wide, broad base than on a narrow wedge, and is also good for hip development. The optimum 'spread-squat' position seems to be protective and curative for those babies born with shallow hip sockets (developmental dysplasia of the hip, DDH). Rates of this condition are lower in cultures that carry in this spread-squat position. Cloth nappies, wide-base slings and the Pavlik harness (a harness worn to correct hip dysplasia) all encourage the flexed, abducted position that is optimal for hip development, locating the femoral head deeply into the socket for full articulation of the joint and encouraging blood supply and growth.

There is controversy and misunderstanding about narrow-based carriers and DDH, so it is worth looking at in a little more depth. The causes of hip dysplasia remain poorly understood. There is an increased risk if there is a positive family history. Female babies seem to be four to five times more at risk than males, and several factors in pregnancy seem to be relevant. For example, reduced amniotic fluid that constricts the baby and prevents free foetal movement, breech birth or another condition that affects how babies lie in utero (such as fixed foot deformity) seem to be related to dysplasia at birth. The left hip seems to be more frequently involved than the right. Furthermore, the growing baby is exposed to the mother's oestrogen hormones. This is thought to be relevant as oestrogen encourages ligament relaxation near the time of delivery, which may help with giving birth. This may also cause laxity in the baby's hip ligaments, increasing the risk of an unstable joint. These are not risks that a parent has any control over. After birth, however, parental choices do have an effect.

Studies strongly suggest that some cultures who swaddle their infants tightly (Native American societies prior to the 1950s, and some Japanese societies) have had a far greater incidence of DDH and childhood hip dislocation. It is interesting to note that when the Najavo Indian culture (where mothers carried their babies tightly bound on cradle boards, with their legs straightened) adopted bulky cloth nappies, the incidence of childhood hip dislocation decreased dramatically, even though they continued to use the cradle boards. The nappies encouraged the babies' legs into a more natural flexed position (like a spread-squat). African cultures, which do not swaddle their babies and carry them constantly on their backs from birth, have a very low incidence of hip dysplasia.

In 2015 the *Journal of Paediatric Orthopaedics* published an article based on data from 40,000 children in Malawi and a systematic review of current evidence:

> 'The majority of mothers in Malawi back-carry their infants during the first 2 to 24 months of life, in a position that is similar to that of the Pavlik harness. We believe this to be the prime reason for the low incidence of DDH in the country. In addition, there is established evidence indicating that swaddling, the opposite position to back-carrying, causes an increase in the incidence of DDH. If a carrying position of infants during their early months of development can reduce the incidence of DDH, then a public health initiative promoting back carrying could have significant world health and financial implications in the future management of DDH and also have potentially huge effects on the timing and severity of development of adult hip arthritis.'[5]

On the whole, babies do not tend to spend prolonged periods in narrow-based carriers (compared to ergonomic ones), so for most children, even with shallow sockets, the risk is low, especially as most DDH is detected early. However, it may be wiser to avoid narrow-based carriers where the legs hang straight down, or full body swaddling, if there is anything in a child's history that could make the condition more likely.

Facing out

Parents often want to carry babies facing the world, as this is what is often seen in the media and among their peers. Babies do enjoy looking around, especially once they are a little older, have mastered head control, and have longer periods awake in the sling. Some families expect to begin carrying babies facing out at this point, and believe that it is the best option for their curious child. Many parents think that babies need to be face out as much as possible for interest and stimulation, rather than looking at their parent all the time. Sometimes this belief is a marker for low self-esteem in a parent; they may worry that they aren't interesting enough, when for many well-attached babies their parent is their most beloved sight. This is especially true if parent and baby are attuned and the parent is responsive and communicative and able to engage happily in play. Babies are often able to pick up on unhappy or uneasy feelings in parents and can be reflexively resistant to close contact, creating a negative spiral. Lots of in-arms carrying, skin-to-skin and time spent together can be very helpful to counter this.

Sometimes babies do resist being carried in a sling facing the parent – this may be because they want to be able to see more if they are very awake, or because they have come to associate the sling with sleeping, which they don't want to do. A parent who is attuned to their child will be more able to work out why a baby is resisting. It could also be a reflection of a disordered attachment relationship brought on by pregnancy or birth trauma for example (please do seek help if this is you!). Maybe the baby does not enjoy the position they are in (straight-down legs being pushed backwards with every parental stride), is feeling too hot, or has reduced visibility. Facing out can seem a solution when in fact most of these issues can be tackled with support.

Before facing a baby away from you, there are some important considerations. Young babies who are perceived to have good head control will still tire easily and their neck muscles fatigue quickly when there is no support in the facing out position, which is literally 'back to front'. A tired baby is less able to 'switch off' and turn into a parent's chest when they have had enough and fall asleep. Manufacturers do not advise sleeping in facing out positions as a heavy head that is unsupported by a parent's chest will droop forwards, with the chin sinking down and putting the chest under slight compression, potentially compromising the airway. A parent who can't see their baby's face or feel their breathing is less likely to be aware of any changes in respiration, and will be slower to react to any problems.

Babies are intensely social creatures and learn to regulate and control their emotions through interaction with their parents. They love to observe their parents' responses, especially to their own actions and noises. If they fail to elicit responses they eventually stop trying to engage and attachment can be harmed. Being able to see a parent's face is vital. Social referencing (triangulation) is very important in the first year and well into the second. It is the mechanism by which a baby learns about the world, based on the response he observes in his trusted parent. Potentially scary experiences can be defused if a baby sees his parent remaining calm, or receives comfort and reassurance. In a structured carrier worn facing out, it isn't as easy for a baby to twist around to see his parent's face. Continual parent-child communication is hampered by facing-away positions. Many pushchair makers now include parent-facing positions as standard, as this is believed to encourage and improve language skills and bonding.

Both parent and baby may be less comfortable than when baby is held facing in, or on the side. The parent's body does not form part of the support structure of the carry when facing out, so much of the work of carrying has to be done by the shoulders, rather than the core postural muscles. Centres of gravity tend to diverge when the baby is held facing out and low down, adding strain to shoulders and back muscles.

Most forward-facing carriers on the market are harness carriers with narrow bases, in which the legs hang straight down, so children tend to be held in straightened positions. This may be less than optimal over a prolonged period, especially when babies are still very young. Some newer carriers create 'bucket seats', almost like little chairs, for babies to sit in more natural positions, supported from knee to knee facing the world. These can be much more comfortable for both parent and child.

The instructions for facing-out carriers usually suggest that the position should only be used for babies over four to five months, for twenty minutes to half an hour at a time. Facing out can be fun for parent and child if done sensitively and thoughtfully, with an eye on the child's anatomical development and comfort.

The period when a baby cannot control his positioning to achieve his desire to see more usually lasts only a few months; with the increased flexibility and coordination that comes with age, they can see more from any position and their frustration decreases. For curious children, there are many comfy options for carrying facing the parent that can still give a baby a good view. Carriers with broadly angled straps that don't get too close to the face can be very useful. As children grow in coordination, they need less head support and often enjoy being 'arms out' (with the panel reaching up to the armpits for safety). It is surprising how far a child can turn round to see when they can move their shoulders! Hip carriers and ring slings will hold a child 'off-centre', or laterally on the hip, giving a wide view, and they will still be able to turn towards their parent for conversation or rest. Back-carrying is another way for a curious child to see the world coming towards them. Most structured carrier makers suggest using this option once your child can sit up, and it is not hard to do on your own. Your local sling library or consultant will be able to help you.

Less structured carriers, which are more mouldable around a baby's body (like woven wraps or mei tais), can be used to back-carry younger children. This can be useful if a parent wants to keep her baby close and safe, but needs the front of her body to be free. The fabric can be tightened strand by strand, and tied carefully to ensure proper back and neck support and that the airway is kept open.

Dressing safely with slings

It is important to make sure that your child is appropriately dressed when in a sling. Body heat is shared when human beings are in close proximity and it is surprising how warm babies are when held on the chest (less so on the back or on the hip). As you warm up (by walking briskly, for example) so will your baby.

Being too hot is not good for babies; it makes them sleepy. Overdressing a baby for bed sleeping is a risk factor for Sudden Infant Death Syndrome (SIDS), so it makes sense to avoid overheating when the baby is sleeping in a sling. Being too bundled up reduces a child's ability to sweat (the drops of sweat need to be able to evaporate to carry heat away), which means even older children can get too hot. It can be surprisingly easy to overheat, as the sling fabric behaves like extra layers of clothing and some padded carriers can become hot. Thick furry snowsuits trap too much warmth to be suitable for use with a sling.

Thick snowsuits pose problems other than overheating. Sometimes the weight of the baby inside the snowsuit means that they sink down inside it, ending up with their faces buried inside the padded fabric. This may be a risk to airway and breathing. The same goes for hooded jackets or thick cardigans that can 'ride up' the back of the carrier. Too much fabric around the chest and upper body will also make it hard to achieve a fully supported carry, with too much space between the baby's head and the parent's chest, allowing his head to slump forwards. Thick fabric (e.g. jeans) can make it hard to achieve a good seat in a carrier. Be aware of your own clothing too; a cowl or a scarf may prove problematic if your small baby snuggles his face into the fabric.

So what is best for keeping warm? Several thin layers are always a good option. Layers trap air in between them, so can be more effective at providing warmth than one or two thick items of clothing. Adding extra layers over you and your baby together (a large shawl, an oversized coat or special babywearing clothing) allows easy undoing or removal if you are getting too warm, without needing to take baby out of the carrier. This also allows parents to remove layers while carrying a sleeping baby from a cold street to the inside of a warm shop, for example, to avoid overheating.

Protecting yourselves from the sun is also important. Choosing cool and lightweight slings can help in hot weather, and some carriers are made of UV-resistant fabric. Exposed heads and limbs can easily burn and adequate hydration is very important.

Umbrellas, waterproof ponchos and hats are useful in wind and rain, and ear defenders can be helpful in outdoor situations where loud noises are likely.

In-arms carrying

There are some clear advantages to in-arms carrying versus using a carrier. Once a baby begins to uncurl and shows signs of wanting to stretch or move, or indicates that he wants to be put down on the floor to explore, this should be respected wherever possible. Babies should to be able to change position and stretch when they need to, and shouldn't be held firmly in the same unchanged position for too long. This lack of movement does not tend to happen with in-arms carrying, as babies are surprisingly strong and wriggly and able to express a clear desire to change their location! A sling, pram or car seat, in contrast, can hold children in relatively static positions for long periods even when they are awake. Obviously sometimes babies need to be transported from one place to another on long journeys, which may mean containing them for longer than is preferable, but this should be kept to a minimum and movement in the container should be encouraged.

If you are using a sling, and baby is contentedly asleep against your body, gently rearranging limbs and turning the head from side to side helps to avoid muscle stress. Babies love to sleep in slings for hours when they are small, and when older they may enjoy being taken for a walk in a sling when there is a lot to look at and fall contentedly asleep after a short while. However, if baby is awake, movement matters. It allows the brain to gather information about proprioception and balance; to engage with the world from an upright position, and should be encouraged. The constant changing of position with in-arms carrying helps with communication and learning and, as babies' vision improves, so does their understanding. If your baby wants to get down and play and it is safe, let her; it is good for her.

In-arms carrying is instinctive for parents; when they begin to ache, they switch arms or move the child to relieve the discomfort. This has the effect of toning different muscle groups and building endurance. Such changes in load bearing are also good for joints and bone health. With a sling, changes of posture and position are often less frequent, as the parent's attention can be engaged elsewhere, so many movement specialists suggest that in-arms carrying is more beneficial than sling use.

Nonetheless, a sling is more comfortable than in-arms carrying for many parents, and carrying is possible for longer. As with any form of exercise, muscles need to get used to greater and more prolonged loading, and I usually recommend gradually increasing the length of time the carrier is used day by day. Some children are heavier than others of the same age or have lower tone; these children can feel harder to carry and a sling can make it easier. It is important to ensure maternal bodies have recovered from pregnancy and that the pelvic floor is in good health before beginning to carry toddlers again – heavy loading for several uninterrupted hours may affect the pelvic floor. Lastly, in-arms carrying is not hands-free, which can be of great importance for simply getting things done.

The important thing is to carry your child in a way that works for you both and allows you to share the world together, bonding and communicating as you go. Listen to your body, carry in many different positions, shift the load about and encourage movement.

The TICKS rules for safe babywearing	
Tight	√
In view at all times	√
Close enough to kiss	√
Keep chin off chest	√
Supported back	√

For the full guidelines, see page 160.

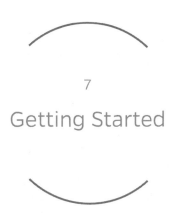

7

Getting Started

So you want to carry your baby, but you're not sure where to start. It is very common to feel overwhelmed by the options, and I strongly recommend that you find your local sling library or consultant and let them help you. They can guide you and allow you to try things out before you buy. Different slings suit different people, and taking advice can help you avoid making a costly purchase that doesn't meet your needs. Below are some general pointers that may be useful.

Safety is of course the most important consideration, and is especially important with young babies who are still small. As we have seen, a baby's airway should be supported by keeping the head well aligned with the spine, avoiding curled-up positions with the chest compressed and chin sunk on to chest. The safest place for a small baby is upright, facing his parent, close enough to kiss, and supported snugly all around to avoid slumping. Ergonomic soft slings and carriers will be respectful to your baby's anatomy, keeping him gently seated in a comfortable position. The close, direct contact will help you to be more aware of your baby's movement and any changes in demeanour or breathing.

Narrow-based harness-style carriers, as we have seen, may not be unsafe when used appropriately for age and size and fitted carefully, but they may not be as comfortable for a baby as the alternatives. They may also be less comfortable for the parent, as they tend not to distribute the weight of the baby around the parent's torso very well. Parents often comment that their backs ache and their babies feel very heavy.

As your baby grows and can hold his head up, his needs will change and how you carry him will change accordingly. Many families find hip and back carrying of great value for babies who want to be able to see more of the world. Toddlers and preschoolers may also need or want to be carried, and there are many slings designed specifically to carry their increased weight.

In summary, choose a sling that supports your child as safely and comfortably as possible and feels enjoyable for you both to wear. Each dyad (parent and child combination) has different preferences and one size does not fit all. A common analogy is trying on shoes; what fits your friend or someone on the internet perfectly may be uncomfortable for you. Some people enjoy tying laces, while others find this harder and prefer zips or buckles. It is all about finding the right combination and everyone will have different priorities (for example, something quick and easy for the school run, versus something more complex but supremely comfortable for long walks).

This is where sling libraries and sling consultants are of great value. They will give you the chance to try different options, then help you make the most of the carrier you choose. They can tweak the fit for maximum comfort, showing you how to use the sling in different ways as your child's needs change, and showing you what to do if it doesn't seem to be working or if your baby doesn't seem to like it.

Stretchy wraps

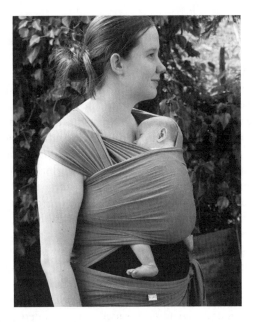

Stretchy wraps come in all shapes and sizes, and are usually seen cuddling a gorgeous tiny baby close to someone's chest, around the house or out on a walk. For many this is the first type of sling they own.

'I'd go out in the morning and T would sleep in the wrap pretty much all day. I'd meet up with other mums or just go and have a coffee and read the paper by myself, without having to worry about manoeuvring a pram.' Alice

'I loved how snuggly it is, closest thing to having my bump back! I loved the way it moulded to him. For a *winter baby it was perfect as it was so warm.'* Janet

A stretchy wrap is a length of fabric, usually made of soft and stretchy machine-knitted cotton, between four and five metres long and about half a metre wide. Some have bamboo fibre blended with the cotton, which adds to the softness and comfort, and some have a small proportion of spandex, which adds to their elasticity and stretch. They are suitable from birth, and in fact are used for kangaroo care of premature babies in hospitals (under careful supervision). Most people find stretchy wraps suitable for at least four to six months and often many more.

Not all stretchy wraps are alike; they vary hugely in quality and supportiveness, but by and large, they have the same purpose – to be a comfortable one-size-fits-most sling that a parent can put on and tie securely before putting baby gently in. Babies are supported by the mouldable fabric in a comfortable, natural seated squat that respects their anatomy and physiology. The gentle stretch often creates a little bit of bounce, which may remind a baby of the movement of his mother walking while he was still in the womb, and the snuggly fabric mimics the gentle all-round pressure he was used to. Babies often sleep well in stretchy wraps, when well positioned, as the closeness and support of the layers of fabric (always use at least two layers of fabric, preferably three) are greatly reassuring. The stretchiness also means that the baby can be quickly removed from the carrier without having to untie it, so the sling can stay on all day and be reused when needed.

Like all carriers, stretchy slings need to be used safely. The most important consideration is to protect baby's airway; a baby's neck should never be folded in half and two fingers should fit between their chin and their chest. The wrap should be tight enough to avoid slumping and can be adjusted to provide head support.

Horizontal 'cradle' carries are no longer recommended by industry professionals, as there is a risk to breathing if a baby's head is pressed forwards onto their chest by fabric behind the head. Forward facing in a stretchy is no longer recommended, even though the practice remains common and some older instruction manuals haven't been updated. Most people think twice before doing a back carry in a stretchy wrap – there are many safety factors to consider and there are other, simpler options for back-carrying.

Some people feel daunted by long lengths of stretchy fabric, but it is really not as difficult as it seems and is easy to learn. After a few goes you will feel more confident. The most common carries are the 'front double hammock carry' and a 'pocket wrap cross carry'. If the ends of the wrap get muddy as they trail on the floor while you tie the stretchy, the wrap can be easily washed. If you prefer less fabric, but like the bounce and snuggliness of the stretchy wrap, a carrier made of slightly stretchy fabric with some structure already built in may be worth trying.

> '*The stretchy is a brilliant hands-free kit. I've been out and about, car seat to wrap, quite a lot. There's an ever so gentle bounce that quickly settles Erin whilst walking around and yet when alert she's still able to have a nosey around. I love babywearing already and find the stretchy very comfortable to carry her 12lb weight.*' Karen

All stretchies are different. The best way to get a feel for them is to try out several at your local sling library; most people prefer two-way stretchies for ease of use.

One-way stretch
Older-style stretchies tend to have what is known as a 'one-way stretch' (they stretch in one direction, usually lengthways).

They are comfortable, but may be harder to get really snug and it will be more tricky to manoeuvre the passes over tiny feet and short legs. Due to the looseness needed to get baby in, they can tend to sag after a period of wear. If you get it right, they can be very supportive as they don't bounce much.

Two-way stretch

Most newer stretchies have varying degrees of 'two-way stretch' (they stretch widthways and lengthways). This often adds a greater degree of manoeuvrability of the passes, and may add a little more elasticity (how easily the wrap will spring back into place after being stretched out to make a pass), which often makes them easier to use than the one-way stretchies. They need to be tied snugly at the start due to their greater stretch, to avoid sagging later. They all feel slightly different, so it is worth trying a few on if you can, or reading unbiased reviews.

Structured stretchy

This is a semi-structured stretchy wrap that has the two cross passes sewn into position, and is tightened once baby is in by pulling any excess fabric through two rings at the side. There is less fabric than the typical stretchy, which some people find useful.

Pouch stretchy

There are some stretchy 'tube' slings – the parent wears two cylinders across the body, one over each shoulder, making two crossed pockets for a baby to sit in, one leg on either side of each tube, with the third tube providing a horizontal pass for back support. They are very simple to put on, but as they come in different sizes, they need to be chosen for the correct fit.

Your baby can rest in the stretchy wrap for as long as he and you are comfortable, with frequent adjustments of position, and feeding/nappy changes as needed. How long your stretchy will last depends on the stretchy and your skills at using it. Some cheaper, lightweight ones feel less supportive as the months go by, while some hybrid stretchies can carry toddlers. Many people find that as babies get bigger and want to be able to see the world ahead of them, they begin to resist facing inwards.

This is the time to investigate different ways of carrying with your stretchy wrap (such as turning the shoulder straps over to provide a greater field of vision), or to move on to a different carrier with greater visibility. Later you may consider carriers that allow off-centre positioning, such as hip carriers like ring slings or buckled hip carriers.

Woven wraps

Woven wraps are sometimes seen as the sling of choice if you want to be a 'real babywearer', in part because of the extra skills required to become very proficient, and also because of the dizzying range of patterns and prices (some can sell for £350 or more). This is unhelpful: *any* parent who chooses to carry their child has made a fantastic choice. It is the carrying and the closeness that confer the huge benefits of physical contact, not the price tag of the sling! Fortunately woven wraps are wonderful, not that hard to master, and don't have to cost the earth.

A woven wrap is wrapped around you and your baby, binding you closely together. The fabric is mouldable, ensuring a snug, smooth fit, and it can be tied to provide excellent support for your baby, and comfortable weight distribution across your body. Wraps are infinitely adjustable and can be tied in many different ways as your baby grows.

Woven wraps have been part of normal family life for countless generations all around the world. Modern woven wraps are long parallelograms of fabric that have been woven on a large loom. The loom is pre-loaded with threads that run vertically (the warp), then another set of threads (the weft) are woven horizontally in and out of the warp threads to create patterns.

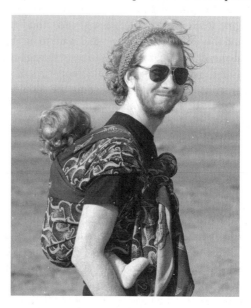

Many woven wraps are still handwoven, and there is a trend towards reviving traditional techniques to preserve cultures and encourage sustainability. However, the majority are now machine-woven. Special techniques to produce and treat the threads ensure the woven wrap has a great deal of strength and durability, making them different from other woven cloths such as tablecloths or clothes. Some are thin, strong and cool to wear, while others are dense and cushy for extra comfort or warmth.

Many parents find wraps the most comfortable type of sling. They do not stretch, and can be carefully tightened in small degrees to create a perfect fit around you and your child. Many young babies enjoy the gentle, consistent all-round pressure and fall asleep during the wrapping process.

> *'It's like a warm, blankety, all-encompassing hug,*
> *moulding to you both perfectly every time.'* Kate

Spreading the wide fabric around your body helps to distribute the weight of your child, and there is great control over positioning and snugness. Fabric can be arranged to ensure even load distribution over the shoulders and avoid digging in, and to ensure children are supported from knee to knee and up to the neck when needed, or to allow arms out for freedom. A woven wrap gives more support than some other carriers for those with back problems, who find they can carry for longer than with other kinds of sling.

Woven wraps are extremely versatile; one wrap can be used from birth to toddlerhood and beyond. One wrap can also be used by more than one person without adjusting the height of straps or buckles, so they can be excellent value for money. Wraps work well for carrying a toddler during pregnancy, or carrying two children together. Hip and back carries can allow high carries for good visibility, so your child can share the world at your eye level, and conversation is easy with a child on your back. Learning these carries does take a little practice. Few people choose to do a facing out carry with a wrap.

> *'I love being able to carry my little one with the wrap,*
> *and when my big child gets tired, it is so useful to be able*
> *to carry him in it too!'* Sarah

Some people prefer not to have long tails of fabric gathering around their feet while putting their child in the sling and choose a shorter wrap. Some enjoy being creative with less fabric, and some families benefit from having a range of carrier styles to choose from. There are no rules!

Wrap fabrics

Most wraps are woven with cotton threads, as cotton is easy to care for, soft, strong and supportive, especially when the thread count is high and the threads are reasonably thick. However, good cotton is not cheap, and the process of creating a wrap is labour-intensive, which explains the price difference between a simple length of cloth and a woven wrap for carrying a child. Some thinner cotton cloths are treated with wax to add extra strength (like African kangas).

Some wraps are woven as blends of cotton with other fibres, such as wool, linen, hemp, silk or bamboo. These fibres can add features such as extra supportiveness, grippiness, softness or glide, and people will often have their own preferences.

For wrapping a newborn, a few qualities are especially valuable, such as softness against tender skin, and a fabric with smoothness and glide during wrapping, to avoid any dragging pressure against baby's back.

- Cotton is among the softest fibres and is very easy to wash, especially if you have a baby who dribbles or possets. Cotton can be combed or treated for extra smoothness and softness.
- Bamboo is also very soft and has a gentle glide, making it lovely to work with. Multi-layer carries tend to work best for carrying bigger children with this fibre.
- Silk is also soft when broken in, but is strong and lightweight which adds longevity. Care may be needed with washing some brands.
- Wool is often bouncy and breathable due to the helical structure of the fibre, and retains warmth well. Wraps with wool can be very soft and are usually quick to break in and easy to wrap with. Newer wool blend wraps are designed to be easy to wash without felting, but caution

is always advised. Some wool can feel prickly on the skin.
- Linen and hemp blends can take a little more work to break in and are often used for carrying heavier children, but once soft and mouldable can be used with newborns.

A little 'grip' is useful to help to 'fix' the carry in place and avoid slipping and sliding, and this can often be gained from the choice of pattern – dense patterns create more friction. Some fabrics are grippier than others, which can affect how easy they are to tighten.

Other factors can affect how a wrap feels, such as how densely the wrap is woven (the thread count, and the looseness of the weave).

Choosing a wrap to use

Woven wraps come in a range of sizes, which are numbered (similar to shoe sizes). Most people start with the standard size 6 (4.6m), which allows most types of carry with most sizes of parent and child. This may be all you need. People often wonder which wrap would be best for a newborn or for a toddler, or for a beginner. I usually advise parents to pick something that they love the look of, and to start with a good, simple cotton wrap, size 6, which is easy to care for. Prices range from £40 upwards.

Stripes can help with learning how to make the passes and which sections to tighten around your baby. Many good brands sell wraps that are soft and ready to use from the first wash, rather than needing a lot of work to soften up (known as 'breaking in').

Most babywearers start with a front carry with a longer wrap for a baby, allowing multiple passes for greater peace of mind. The classic front wrap cross carry is ideal, as this is simple, supportive to small bodies and respectful of physiology. It is not hard to learn and easy to adjust. There are many good videos and tutorials available, and any good sling librarian or consultant should be able to show you how to do it safely and comfortably, protecting baby's airway and supporting their hips and spine.

The type of carry you choose to use can change frequently depending on the needs of your child; light snuggly front carries in the early baby days, other front, hip or back carries as they grow, single-layer cooler carries, multi-layer carries for warmth or greater support; a woven wrap allows all these variations.

Wraps are therapeutic

It may seem like a minor point, but the attractiveness of woven fabrics can be very therapeutic, especially if clothing choices in parenthood have become restricted. Colour therapy is believed to lift the mood, and a pretty wrap can sometimes help with motivation to get out and about for a walk with your child, or look very special at a celebration. There is an incredible range of patterns to choose from, be it stylishly classy, or a riot of exuberant colour. Life with a small baby can be challenging, and many parents enjoy the opportunity to learn a new set of skills with their woven wraps, experimenting with carries, the feel of different fabrics and perfecting their technique. This can become a sociable activity.

'I love the versatility of a wrap but I've also found it really interesting learning about the technical side of things – experiencing different fabrics and how they perform differently, practising new carries, recognising different companies' styles.' Lindsay

'The effort is worth it for me because being unable to breastfeed left me worried I would struggle to bond. Wrapping gives me precious bonding and closeness, and gives my daughter the ability to experience the world from a position of total security. It makes us feel like a team.' Jodie

Asian-style carriers

A mei tai is the common name given to a type of Asian carrier that originated in China, made of a fabric panel with long straps that are wound around the parent's body, to be tied or twisted or tucked away securely. The Chinese name for this type of carrier has become eponymous for the style, but different cultures have their own variants of these cloth carriers.

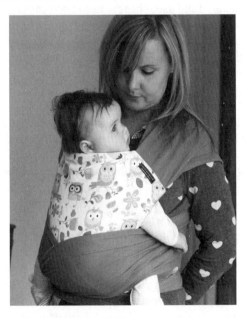

Mei tai styles of carrier have been made from many different fabrics, from reeds and grasses to woven cloths covered with beads. Many are beautifully made and display painstaking cultural craftsmanship, yet are extremely practical for daily life. Most modern variants are made from cotton or canvas and some are made from woven wraps. They have been the inspiration for many current Western slings, including the modern buckled carriers.

In the Western world, mei tais are popular with those who appreciate the mouldability and support of woven wraps but prefer something with more structure than a length of fabric. It can be easier to secure a child quickly with a mei tai. Some prefer the flexibility and adjustability of the mei tai to the more structured and fixed shape of full-buckle carriers. As the straps are wrapped around and knotted, they can be tightened and adjusted to fit around the body exactly, which can be more of a challenge with some buckle carriers, which are limited by the placement of buckles or the length of webbing.

A mei tai consists of a fabric panel that has two straps at the base that are tied (or buckled, in some variants) securely around the waist, and two straps from the top of the panel that can be wrapped around the parent's shoulders and across baby to ensure a snug and comfortable fit. Baby sits in the pouch created by the panel with their legs out on either side, and the long straps allow a great degree of adjustability to all shapes and sizes. Some are made of simple cotton, others are converted from woven wraps.

Broad, slightly padded straps are more comfortable than thinner, narrower straps which don't distribute the weight as well. Wide straps made from wrap fabric are popular as they can be spread across the wearer's shoulders and wrapped around baby's bottom for extra lift and support.

Some mei tais have padded waistbands, while others have none; it is all a question of personal preference.

'I adore my wrap conversion mei tai because it is simply the best of both worlds. It has the easy ups of a full-buckle carrier, but all the beauty and floppy comfort of a wrap. Wrap straps offer extra support across my baby's bum and

spread the weight more across the shoulders so we are super comfy... And we can't forget, it's full of sleepy dust!' Emily

Mei tais can be worn on the hip with bigger babies, to give them a wider viewpoint, and can also be worn on the back. As they are so adjustable, the long straps can be tied to extend the width of the carrier, ensuring your bigger child has a good, wide seat for longer than they would do in a full-buckle carrier. On the whole, babies are not carried facing out in mei tais.

'*I love carrying my toddler in our mei tai. There are some days where nothing will do but Mummy, and with a sling she gets the closeness she needs and I can still get things done. It's also invaluable for special occasions which often get overwhelming for her. This way she can feel safe and secure and we get to spend more time as a family. Part of the reason I love mei tais so much is because they are half-way between wrapping and buckles, the ease and speed of buckles with the support and versatility of wrapping'.* Hannah

'*I love mei tais. They offer some of the structure and ease of use of buckle carriers, but with an added ability to mould to the shapes of me and my little boy. For me, there's also something about tying rather than buckling the straps that appeals both in terms of aesthetics and wearability. Versatile, and wonderfully comfortable – I get such joy and closeness from carrying my little one in this way.'* Anna

Variants of mei tais

There are several variants of the basic mei tai which can add extra useful features. 'Half-buckles' are mei tais with buckled waists but long shoulder straps for tying (this can be useful if you feel uncertain which knot to untie first to get baby out!). 'Onbuhimos' have rings at the waistband for the long straps to be threaded through, and work especially well for back carries. 'Podaegis' have two straps at the top of a long blanket. The straps are tied around parent and baby the same way as a mei tai and can be used on the front or the back. There is no waistband on either of these carriers, which can be useful if you are pregnant and carrying your toddler. South Korean 'chunei' carriers are similar to jackets fastened around the parent's body that have a pocket for baby to sit in.

Full-buckle carriers

The full-buckle carrier is the 'modern' version of more ancient carrying methods, taking advantage of newer sewing and padding techniques as well as the development of plastic buckles and webbing. It is the most popular style of carrier for today's parents and they are usually made of cotton or canvas, woven fabrics or polycotton breathable fabrics. Full-buckles have a structured panel, often a waistband, and two shoulder straps that buckle together to hold the child close to the carer's body. Good full-buckle carriers are designed to keep baby snugly close and high up (close enough to kiss) and ensure the airway is protected for safe breathing. They should ensure the spine is held gently in the natural curve with the knees above the bottom, supporting them gently from the kneepits up to the back of the head (with head support if needed). Carriers like this are usually very comfortable for the caregiver, and children are often carried contentedly well into the toddler years and beyond.

There are many variants on the basic model, such as the type and structure of the waistband, the way the straps fasten (cross straps or rucksack straps), and the height and width of the panel. Generalisations such as 'you need a carrier with a

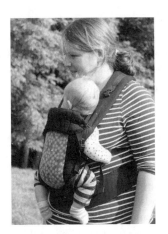
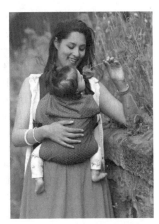

waistband for support if you have back pain', or 'you'd be better off with a carrier that crosses the straps if you want to front carry' can be unhelpful. Each parent-child dyad is unique and it is all about how each carrier distributes the weight around the body, which varies enormously from parent to parent.

On the whole, most buckle carriers fit babies from three months upwards, and stretchy or woven wraps and ring slings are more useful with newborns. However, there are a few full-buckle carriers that can be used safely and comfortably from birth. Some have inbuilt support structures for babies of 7lb and upwards, while some have adjustable back panels that can be rolled up and narrowed to fit, or foldable sections that snap into place to reduce the size and width of the carrier.

Many other carriers have separate inserts to make the volume inside the panel smaller and babies perch on the insert in seated postures. These can be very useful but also a bit fiddly to get right with especially small babies and some work better than others. Most people find that they enjoy buckle carriers most once their small babies have grown a little bit stronger, with more muscle tone and a little bit of head control.

The facing-in towards caregiver position is the most favoured; this allows good airway, spine and hip support, as well as being a safe position to sleep in when needed – many babies love to sleep in the sling close to parent's chest, just as they would in arms. This facing-in position keeps the baby and caregiver's centres of gravity as close together as possible, and can allow active social referencing (when a baby experiences something in her field of vision and is able to turn to see what her caregiver makes of the same experience). This allows the baby to assess and process a new experience in the light of her caregiver's response ('This person is nice, we can smile at him', versus 'That dog is worrying, I should be cautious.').

If you have an active baby who wants to see the world, a carrier with a broad upper section will allow good movement of baby's arms and head for a wide field of vision, and allow older babies to get an elbow out to turn their shoulders around. There are hip buckle carriers which can allow the best of both worlds (good visibility, good position, good opportunities for social referencing, and good comfort too!)

Full-buckles are very popular for back carrying bigger children once they can sit up and have excellent head control (although many parents continue to front carry beyond six months), as this allows children the chance to see where they are going and gives parents the freedom to explore further afield, or care for new babies more easily.

'Our buckled carrier is the perfect tool for winding down for bedtime on a camping trip, resting tired little legs whilst hiking (without the bulk of a framed carrier), and elevating her out of danger in busy, crowded areas.' Tricia

'I love my buckle. It is quick and easy to use, especially

in the rain on school runs, and it is super comfy when it is adjusted well and fits properly.' Laura

'I find them so much easier to use than fabric slings because of the mobility problems with my hands.' Alex

'Buckles are dad and family friendly and convenient for toddlers who are up and down all day.' Andrew

'They are easy to buy from mainstream sellers and can come in so many gorgeous prints.' Harriet

Hip carriers

Hip carriers can be very useful for parents who have children who want to see more of the world, but aren't ready for back carries and want to preserve the visual connection of parent-facing positions. They come in fabric carriers (ring slings – usually made of woven wrap fabric for extra comfort and support – and pouches, often made of sturdy cotton), some buckled carriers and a few 'carrying aids' that are not hands free.

Ring slings are beautiful and versatile carriers that suit many families. They are great with younger babies, for curious bigger babies for short periods of time, and for toddlers wanting quick up-and-downs.

'We love how convenient it is. You can just pop him in and go. It's the easiest way of doing short journeys where you're taking him in and out lots. If I could only have one sling, it'd be a ring sling.' Carla

A ring sling is a piece of woven fabric, usually about 2m long and 60cm wide, that has one end sewn securely into two strong rings. The rings should be circular single-piece non-welded metal rings with no sharp edges, for safety reasons. Plain cotton ring slings with thick plastic rings are often harder to get snug and may not be as comfortable.

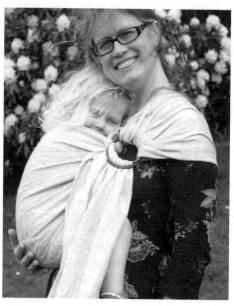

They are worn on one shoulder with your child sitting in a pouch on the opposite side of your body, with the loose end of the fabric threaded through the rings in such a way that the tension holds the fabric firmly and the weight is distributed across your shoulder and back. The child is in the spread-squat position, with the lower third of the fabric providing a hammock seat to hold them securely.

Ring slings are versatile for a wide age range and can pack away small, which is convenient. Once you have the knack, they are very quick and easy to put on. They can be used from birth, and allow the natural foetal curved position with knees tucked up. Many babies sleep contentedly in a ring sling, allowing the carrying parent to be hands free. Ring slings are useful for feeding as they can provide discreet cover, or allow semi-cradled or sideways seated positions for breast or bottle access, as long as the chin remains off the chest. They can be perfect for quick up-and-downs with toddlers, or to keep in the car for emergency carrying needs. They can also be used for back carries for older babies, with care and practice.

> 'I love being able to just pop it in my bag and always have it around for emergencies, whether they be a toddler that can't walk another step or a baby that just needs to be close.' Emily

> 'When he was little, it was such a cosy way to carry him, cuddled in close. When he was a bit bigger, he was too curious for other carriers, and would only sit on our hips – so the ring sling was all we used for a couple of months.' Jemma

> 'I see parents of kids the same age struggling to maintain a hip carry with their child needing to hang on too, but H can snuggle down for a safe doze in the ring sling and my hands are free.' Tricia

There are several different types of ring slings. Some can be bought ready-made, while others are converted from woven wraps by seamstresses. If in doubt, do ask for advice. The fabric used is personal preference, such as 100 per cent cotton, or cotton blended with other fibres to add extra supportiveness. There are also different types of shoulders; a gathered shoulder (which spreads widely to cup the shoulder and upper back) or a pleated shoulder (which can sit more neatly but may spread less). People find they have preferences, so it is worth trying a few out if you can at your local sling library.

Simpler than ring slings but very similar, pouches are 'tubes' of non-stretchy fabric, usually cotton, which are folded in half along their length and then partly unfolded to make a deep pouch for baby to sit in. You need the right size for your body shape for them to work well, so they do need to be fitted and used properly. They can be risky if used badly, as it is very easy for a young baby to slip down inside the pouch and end up with the chin pressed on to the chest or their face squashed against the parent. That said, once a baby is nearer four months or so, with robust upper body control, pouches can be very useful for quick carries as they pack down so small.

There are a few buckled hip carriers that support children fully and are hands free; many parents find them invaluable tools for getting on with daily life with a child held comfortably on the hip, leaving their front free for tasks or caring for other children.

Carrying aids are not technically slings at all, as they are not hands-free. They do not support a child knee to knee and up to the neck, and the parent will need to use an arm to keep the carried child steady. Shaped mesh cross-body sashes balance a child on the hip with some of the weight borne by the opposite shoulder, and small shaped seats buckle around the parent's waist for a child to perch on. Both types need a steadying hand to prevent a child arching back.

With all one-shouldered carriers, it is important to build up strength and ensure frequent changes of position and, if possible, swap sides to encourage balancing of load around the body and avoid strain from repetitive weight bearing that feels comfortable at the time. For safety, the pouch of all hip carriers must be fully adjustable to hold baby snugly all around, with no loose edges; your local sling professional will be able to advise. Once this has been mastered, hip carriers are an excellent option for many.

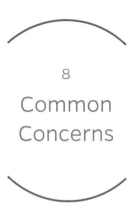

8

Common
Concerns

In this section we will look at some of the most common concerns that people have when they begin to use a sling.

Do slings create clingy children?

Many parents worry that by carrying their baby, specifically in a sling rather than in arms, they are going to create a 'clingy child' who won't be put down. It is disconcerting for a mother who has carried her child frequently from birth to find that he wants to be held much more than his contemporaries, and when the time comes (if it does) for childcare from other individuals, her baby may protest vigorously and not allow another adult to look after him.

All too often parents are told that they have made a rod for their own backs. Doubts can creep in; parents fear that somehow, somewhere, a wrong choice has been made and their child's independence has suffered. Bystanders who see parents and children struggling to separate may think that sling use is more trouble than it is worth.

However, consider what we know about the value of close bonding and attachment. If a child has been carried in arms or a sling from birth, as is the biological norm, and has strong, secure bonds with his caregivers, it is entirely expected and natural for the child to protest when he is removed from his trusted habitat and asked to accept different caregivers he may not know. This child is not 'clingy' in the sense our society means it; he is simply habituated to the close contact he has enjoyed all his life, just as his ancestors were. Babies do become habituated very easily; to breastfeeding, to a dummy, to a favourite blanket with its particular scent. With the natural progression of a child's emotional and psychological development, as well as the growth of his physical skills and strength, he will need and want to be carried less and less, and will rely on it less and less, if his other needs are met appropriately. Until that stage is reached, a child will expect continuity of care in the way he has always experienced it.

Significant changes in circumstances will drive a child to find security where he is used to finding it; in his parents' arms, where he has always found it before. The eight month to twelve month period is often when children experience separation anxiety and this often coincides with parents returning to work and the introduction of new spaces and places. The sling can play a part in providing reassurance, rather than being the root of any 'clinginess'. In contrast, some babies who have been carried much less and put down a lot more may appear to separate from their parents earlier, but for some this will come at a cost in terms of secure attachments.

Carried babies who want to be carried beyond the 'fourth trimester' are babies enjoying normal biological parenting; but as this is very different from the present societal norm, it is perceived as inappropriate and delaying independence. This begs the question, when does normal, biological independence for the human child develop? Anthropological studies suggest this would be when a child has completely self-weaned from breastfeeding and bed-sharing, no longer requests frequent in-arms carrying, is able to reliably move from place to place unaided, and is able to verbally communicate effectively. This begins from around age three for carrying (breastfeeding and bedsharing often continue for much longer in less Westernised cultures). It is worth bearing this in mind when we think about what we expect of our year-old babies.

In our present culture, babies are actively expected and encouraged to be independent early on. Children are incredibly adaptive, and there is a huge array of technology available to encourage early independence, including nightlights, white noise toys and so on. Babies can and do learn to separate from their parent sooner than they normally would. They can learn not to raise their arms or cry for contact, they can learn to stop asking for breastmilk, and they can learn to sleep alone. However, we should be wary of depriving them of the opportunity for the emotional and psychological growth that all these things can offer.

It is no surprise that when a parent chooses a more instinctive and natural means of childrearing, they sometimes clash with other parents and the older generation. Many families feel they have little choice about how much time they spend with their children; regret or resentment about this may manifest itself as criticism when others are able to arrange their lives to allow this. Grandparents may feel rejected if their own children choose to parent differently. Also, when people are confronted by something unfamiliar, they may feel the need to assert themselves by making comments that aren't based on genuine observation. This can create tension. Gentle discussion about current research and our new knowledge of child development, and tactful understanding, can go a long way towards resolving conflicts.

People often worry that their babies will only ever sleep in a sling or resting on them. This is the natural, normal place for a child to sleep, where he feels warm, safe and loved. As babies grow, their need to sleep in-arms gradually declines. If you have the kind of life that cannot allow a child's sleep physiology to mature at its natural pace, then it would be wise to ensure that your baby is well used to happily and easily and trustingly settling to sleep in different locations. This will be easier if he has well-established underlying attachment foundations, and parents who respond to his needs as they arise. All children eventually learn to feed themselves, settle themselves to sleep, walk unaided and accept care from other adults; some learn it sooner than others.

As parents to vulnerable little people who cannot make choices themselves, it is our responsibility to choose a method of childrearing that feels right to us, is the most helpful for our children and is the best that we can do in the circumstances that we live in. Sometimes such choices require sacrifice and a willingness to reconsider our previously held ideas. Choosing to be counter-cultural can be uncomfortable, but can also be very rewarding if based on solid foundations. If a sling feels right to you, use it as much as you and your child wish.

Breastfeeding in slings

Many mothers are able to feed their babies in slings, from the breast or from the bottle, and this can be very a useful skill.

Mums of more than one child often appreciate being able to feed the baby on the go. This is especially true if they are practising responsive feeding, which means acting on a baby's early hunger cues, and have an older child who needs their parent just as much. These mothers have often had some experience of breast or bottle-feeding already, and may be very familiar with their sling, finding it easy to combine the two skills. Mums of older children who can feed quickly in a sitting upright position may also find a sling an invaluable and very convenient tool for getting on with daily life. Parents of small babies may use a sling to carry their child to a place where they can be taken out to feed in peace and comfort. For others, having baby supported partly with the sling and partly with one arm may allow some simple multi-tasking. For others, the extra support of the sling can actually make positioning for feeding easier and become an aid while navigating a tricky breastfeeding journey.

On the whole, it's helpful to consider each element – feeding, and using the sling – as a separate skill to master. When both are confidently mastered, they may be able to be combined. Practice will, of course, be needed!

All the basic rules of sling safety apply when feeding in a sling. As always, protecting the airway and ensuring breathing is unobstructed are of paramount importance.

Babies, on the whole, are obligate nasal breathers. This means that they find it much easier to breathe through their noses than their mouths for the first few months of life, and it is essential that noses are kept clear of any obstruction. This is why babies are able to feed for prolonged periods without needing to delatch, and why those with mild snuffly respiratory infections affecting the small nasal passages may struggle to breathe while feeding.

While a baby's mouth is engaged with sucking and swallowing, his only patent airway is his nose, so it is important for the carer to be consciously aware of any potential obstruction, either external (from sling fabric, breast tissue, or clothing) or internal (neck bent over too far) and to act quickly if required.

Whether feeding upright, or slightly reclined, the safest positions are:

- those in which the parent is actively engaged
  and frequently checking on their child, and able to

recognise any changes
- those that ensure a good air supply at all times with no fabric over the head and chin off the chest (check you can fit two fingers underneath if you are unsure)
- those in which baby's head is aligned with his spine and only turned slightly to one side if needed
- those in which baby's back and occiput (lower part of the back of the head) are appropriately supported
- those in which baby's knees are above the bottom and hips are flexed
- those that ensure that a baby who has finished feeding or has fallen asleep is returned to the most optimal upright position to keep the airway supported and open.

The choice of best position will vary from person to person, depending on the individual circumstances, but the majority of successful 'on-the-go' feeding is done in the upright position. Breastfeeding in horizontal carrying positions needs to be done with great caution. If baby is held face inwards with the sling fabric pulled up over the back of the head, the face will be pushed into breast tissue. This is risky, especially for a snuffly baby, who would be unable to delatch as the head is not free. Babies who fall asleep at the breast in the sling should never be left to sleep in feeding positions, as their disproportionately heavy heads can easily droop or be folded over, with subsequent obstruction of their airways. A little rearrangement is vital.

To make breastfeeding in a sling as easy as possible, think about ensuring easy access for your baby. Your choice of clothes can help. Consider loose-fronted tops that can easily be moved out of the way, or those that open and close with zips or poppers, rather than buttons. Many mums swear by a combination of a loose shirt that can be lifted up/pulled down with a stretchy camisole or vest. Bras that are easy to undo one-handed (while your other hand supports baby's head) are also helpful. Some mums find latching on more successful if they lean forward slightly to bring the breast up to baby's mouth (once breastfeeding is well established), and many need to hold their breast up with one hand for the duration of the feed. Hoods can help with providing some discreet coverage, but remember that temperatures inside slings rise quickly if air cannot circulate freely, and carbon dioxide levels in rebreathed air are raised.

It is possible to feed a baby in most types of sling, with a bit of care. Completely hands-free feeding can't be achieved, as one hand or arm should always be on your baby to provide support, especially before they have excellent head control. But one hand free is better than none! Breast size, shape, flexibility and nipple position vary from woman to woman, and from stage to stage in the breastfeeding journey, so each dyad will need practice to work out which height works best for them. Larger breasts may prove more tricky for some.

Stretchy and woven wraps can be used for feeding, by loosening the fabric slightly to allow baby's position to be altered. Ring slings can be loosened at the rings a little to lower baby to the point at which the nipple is accessible. Buckles and ties from soft structured carriers can also be loosened off to provide access. All types of sling should be retightened, and baby repositioned, when feeding is finished.

In general, many people manage to feed happily and safely in slings, once they are armed with good information and know what to watch out for. It often works best with older children. If you feel unsure about feeding your child in your carrier, do get in touch with a professional who can give you some one-to-one help and advice.

Crying in slings

'*My child cries in the sling… she seems to hate being put into it…*'

This is a frequent concern for parents trying out a carrier for the first time – either the very first sling they have ever used, or when trying to find something more suitable or comfortable for their child's needs as well as their own. Many parents worry that their child hates the carrier they have spent money on, or are convinced that there is no sling out there that will suit their baby. However, it is very common for babies and toddlers to fuss and cry and wriggle in slings. The key is to try to understand the child's experience – to put yourself in their shoes (or booties!)

Babies are small people with feelings just like those of adults, but lacking language they express these feelings through more limited means – laughing, wriggling, crying, bouncing, sucking, moaning, yelling, chewing, rooting, leaning, twisting and so on. Being able to read and understand your baby's cues is vital to a good relationship and this is one of the benefits of a carrier; parents and carers are usually much more aware of and rapidly responsive to a child who is close to their bodies. It is good that your baby is protesting – they are communicating with you and you know it! Now you need to meet the need your baby is expressing and thereby solve the problem. The sling itself may not be the cause of the baby's displeasure.

- Is your baby too hot? It is common for babies to quickly get very warm in a sling. We all know it's unpleasant to be sweaty and over-dressed.
- Is your baby thirsty or hungry? It is always worth making sure your baby is well fed before you embark on a new experience. Most sling professionals will be more than happy for you to feed your baby at sessions – you are more likely to be able to absorb information when your child is happy. You can talk while feeding and you can always to try the carrier again later.

Bringing a baby close to breasts full of milk often creates a desire to be fed, or to suck, even if tummies are full. If you were a baby who could smell milk, and you were being held in a position where you couldn't reach it, you might kick, or wriggle, or yell, so always try offering a feed before trying the carrier again.

- Does your baby feel too full to tolerate pressure on his tummy, like an adult after a large meal? A seated sideways carry may be more comfortable.
- Is your baby wet or dirty, or need to eliminate? Babies are very aware of their own bodily functions.
- Is your baby tired? Many babies have a fussy period before they go to sleep. You may already be aware of this tendency in bed, in the car or in the pram, and a sling is no different. A baby may learn that slings mean sleep, and if he doesn't wish to sleep, he may protest. A little rocking with baby in the sling or a short walk outside is usually enough to help them drift off. Sometimes the new experience of trying a sling can be too much stimulation for a weary baby, pushing him over the edge from tiredness to tantrum, just as it would if you tried to feed him, or change his clothes.
- Is your baby in pain? Teething can be uncomfortable; distraction by play is a great tool, and if a baby suddenly has less distraction he may become aware once again of the ache in his jaws. Abdominal distension from constipation or sore genitalia may also affect carrying.
- Is your baby responding to how she is being handled? Activating primitive reflexes can make babies feel insecure and unwilling to settle into a sling. Lifting and holding your baby securely but gently, from both the upper body and below the bottom, can help to calm them. Being able to support baby confidently

while you bring the carrier up around them will also build their trust. Practice will help.

- Is your baby responding to how you feel? If you are anxious or irritable, your baby will pick up on your muscle tone, shaky breathing and jerky movements and become distressed as something feels wrong. Sometimes it is better to just try again later when you are in a better frame of mind.

- Could you and your baby have some difficulties connecting, perhaps due to a complex pregnancy or a traumatic birth history? Unspoken feelings about how your child arrived in the world can significantly affect bonding, as can prolonged separation in the first few days or weeks of life. The rate of post-traumatic stress disorder after birth is surprisingly high (up to 9 per cent) and there are studies that demonstrate that such stress can impair bonding.[1] Babies are very sensitive to the feelings of their carers and will react accordingly – your baby's behaviour and distress could be a signpost to some of your own internal discord and pain. Midwives, postnatal doulas and the NHS Afterthoughts services can be very helpful, guiding families to find resolution and healing.

Your baby's personality is also important. I often meet people who expect their babies to become utterly still in a sling, and to remain very calm. After all, they're being carried close now, in a giant hug. What's not to love? What's not to be happy about? Well, not everyone appreciates all-over cuddles, especially if they're not tired, or if they want to be active. This is when understanding your baby's personality is useful. Imagine that you are playing happily. All of a sudden you are lifted up and wrapped knee to neck in a giant warm bandage, or suddenly put into a carrier. Perhaps you can't see out very well. Some babies love this and settle down in happy drowsiness (usually because they are ready for cuddles, or are familiar with a well-loved sling). Others may enjoy the sudden change of height and scenery and being able to smell their carer. Still others may feel annoyed at being taken away from their activity, be cross about not being able to see, or feel too hot… these babies may strain and bounce and wriggle or cry in protest. Most children I meet are pretty active in some way – and it is unreasonable to expect them to suddenly change from an active, inquisitive personality to a more docile, still and placid one, especially if the parent also stands strangely still, with their muscles tense with anxiety about the use of the carrier and whether the baby will like it.

Getting your baby into a sling with ease

Being familiar with your sling before you start is helpful. Sling libraries and sling consultants are usually well stocked with weighted demo dolls, which allow you to figure out how to use the sling safely and confidently. If you are very unsure while using the carrier, your baby will pick up on your nervousness and become unsettled. This applies to every kind of carrier. Practice, even with a teddy, and in front of a mirror, will really help, as can videos recommended by your local professional. Preparation (for example, knowing how to keep a child high on your body while you bring the panel up smoothly, or having a ring sling already set up) can make a world of difference to the speed at which you can get the carrier on, before your baby gets fed up.

You can engage your baby during the process. If baby is happily playing, respect that and don't just snatch her away. Offering a well-chosen toy or necklace can help engage a child, as can talking or singing to her. Tell her what you are doing and make the process of being put into the carrier enjoyable in its own right. Rock or sway while you go through each step, and take your time – there is no reason why you can't stop halfway through to show your baby her reflection in the mirror, for example.

- Observe how your baby likes to be carried in-arms. Does she prefer hip carries? Does he love piggy backs? Try to reproduce this as far as you can. Babies are often 'nosy' in the four to eight month period, and ring slings or buckle hip carriers can be a brilliant way to carry a baby to meet their need to be inquisitive! Their preferences will often change as they grow.
- Check your baby is safe (keeping his airway open and his breathing unobstructed is vital).
- Check that he is comfortable – if something feels wrong or hurts him, he will let you know somehow. Understanding how to create a comfortable position that allows deep relaxation is important. We all shift our positions without thinking during the day (re-crossing legs, pulling up socks) and it is hard for a baby to do this as easily. We must be caring and careful. Familiarise yourself with the ideal M-shape position (knees above bum with pelvis tilted inwards), which will avoid any strain on the joints and allow a comfortable curve of the spine. A shift from a 'splatted starfish' position to a hammock-shaped seat can really help a baby's enjoyment of a sling. Ensure baby can move her legs freely at the knee (make the carrier narrower if needed), and check no red marks are developing (raising the knees can help). Babies' hands should have free and easy access to their mouths for sucking or exploring. Check that fabric is not digging into baby's neck and that any knots, webbing or buckles are not pressing on baby's body.

Ensure baby feels secure, but not restrained or restricted.

Remember that your baby still wants to experience the world even while carried, as they do when playing on your lap or on the floor. Help them to be able to see a little, in a way that is appropriate for their age and respectful of growing spines and hips. A carrier that has straps or fabric that comes close to the face may be irritating (remember that babies grow taller, and many carriers can be adjusted to ensure faces and heads are not obscured). If they have good head control, careful arms out can really help with baby's enjoyment. Make sure that there is some activity going on – we all know about the sway we do to settle babies when carried in arms, and how often we shift them around, or the rocking/pushing of the pram – this gives a child some sensory input. It is often worth going for a short walk when you have just put your baby in a sling – the motion and movement, fresh air and change of scenery usually work wonders and you come back with a happier baby. Of course, once you stand still again baby may protest!

Learning a new skill takes a little time and effort… for you and your baby. New experiences need to be absorbed and processed. Every day is a new day, and we all have off days! If you use your carrier a little bit every day, for walks or participating in safe but engaging activities, bit by bit it will get easier and your baby happier. The more relaxed and confident you are, the more your baby will respond to that. Don't force it: take your cue from your baby! If, after a fair shot at it, things still don't feel right, try another carrier from your local sling library and ask a consultant/peer supporter to check your positioning.

Sleeping in slings

Imagine you are a very tired parent, with a new baby who doesn't seem able to settle in their Moses basket or cot, and will only sleep when held and rocked. Your baby cries when he is laid down, no matter how deeply he seemed to be asleep on your chest or your partner's shoulder. This is when you might turn to a baby carrier, which keeps your baby close, in the supported position she loves, able to hear your heartbeat and breathing.

So far so good: your baby is positioned well in the sling, her airway is protected, breathing is unobstructed, spine and head are well aligned with a supported upper back and a gentle curve into a tilted pelvis with an M-shape. Your baby's face is visible and she is close enough to kiss; there is no slumping. Your rocking movements (swaying, walking) and precious closeness have worked their magic, and your baby is peacefully and contentedly and finally asleep.

At this point, the relief is enormous. The temptation is very, very strong, to just sit down in a cosy armchair and close your eyes, or to have a little lie down on the bed well propped up with pillows. The trouble is that one of the central tenets of safe babywearing is to be aware of your baby at all times. Safety reminders aim to protect your baby's airway and breathing, and the only way you can monitor this is by being alert. It doesn't take long for a baby's breathing to become compromised, and the risk is greatest in babies under four months old, whose heads are disproportionately large and heavy and who have not yet developed the strength to support themselves. A sleeping baby's head can roll forward on to their chest, which is also slightly compressed. This is why head support is so vital, and why a baby's face must be visible at all times. Studies have shown that forward lolling of the head can cause desaturation (reduced levels of oxygen in the blood).[2] Another study has shown that babies asleep in the optimal upright position, with chin up and the head well supported on the parent's chest, do not show clinically significant desaturations.[3] It is safe for a baby to sleep upright in a sling if the appropriate guidelines are followed.

A sleeping parent, however, will not be able to check their baby's position and correct any breathing difficulties. Grunting, snoring or other unusual noises should always prompt a check on your baby's position, and it is hard to be aware of such changes when you are almost or fully asleep. Your body position changes as your muscles relax in sleep. Your arms may move and slide apart if you are just holding your baby. If your baby is in a sling, the sling may not remain tight and supportive. Your baby may slump over or curl up into a ball with his chin on his chest, or roll to one side. You may roll over as you relax and unwittingly place too much pressure on parts of your baby's body, or encourage him to roll with you.

If you have had something alcoholic to drink, are a smoker, are on medications that could make you drowsy, or have a medical condition that could impair your ability to be aware of your child at all times, you may wish to reconsider how you are caring for your baby when you are tired. In short, if you are asleep, you are unaware of what you and your baby are doing.

There are of course some ways that a short nap can be done safely with your baby asleep in your arms or in a carrier. For example, your partner could remain in the room with you, and be alert while you and baby enjoy a rest together, in a slightly-reclined, well supported position that ensures baby is still upright. If you are in hospital with your premature baby and are encouraged to share skin-to-skin contact inside a simple stretchy wrap or kangaroo care shirt or boob tube or under a blanket, you may nod off in the chair. You and your baby will be very closely monitored throughout, and chairs often recline at special angles to make it easy for a baby to rest chest to chest, with head well supported.

So, is it safe for a parent to sleep while their child is in a sling? This is a decision for each parent to make, armed with information, with their focus on their child's safety.

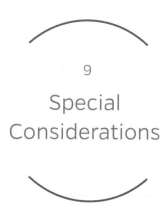

9

Special
Considerations

Carrying in the post-partum period

Babies want to be held close from the very moment they enter the outside world; they crave contact and many will spend their first few days sleeping in their parents' arms and feeding frequently, enjoying this close interaction.

Pregnancy can be tiring and uncomfortable, partly due to our changing bodies and habits. We are no longer an upright species but a sedentary one, to our great anatomical and physiological disadvantage; chronic pain is a significant problem for increasing numbers of people in our society. Symphysis Pubis Dysfunction (SPD) can be debilitating for pregnant women, and there is a growing concern that many women's bodies are not in optimal condition to carry a child, and thus take longer to recover from pregnancy than would have been true of our forebears. Ligament softening and laxity (from the hormonal changes preparing a body to deliver a baby) can take some time to resolve fully, especially if there has been pre-existing back pain and poor posture, and breastfeeding may prolong the effects of relaxin.

Labour, while exhilarating and empowering for some, can be exhausting for others, especially if prolonged. The recent historical practice of lying down for delivery is in marked contrast to how most women around the world across history and cultures have given birth (upright, squatting or kneeling). The natural birth movement and the emergence of doulas to support women's delivery choices mirror a desire to get back to our ancient human roots, which may also encourage speedier recovery from labour and birth.

The rate of caesarean sections (both planned and emergency) is high in Western society. In the UK caesareans account for 20–25 per cent of births (with some regional variation). A caesarean is major abdominal surgery and recovery time varies enormously from woman to woman, depending on the reasons for the operation. Women are advised to avoid heavy lifting, 'carry nothing heavier than your baby', and not to drive for at least six weeks after birth. Scars can be uncomfortable and slow to heal, and some may experience abdominal pain for a while afterwards.

In this context it is not surprising that mothers worry that they may not be strong or well enough to carry their newborns in their arms for prolonged periods. Many will also have toddlers at home, needing the reassurance of their mother's loving arms to help them cope with the newcomer's arrival. Paternity or parental leave is often short; after a few weeks mothers are often required to manage at home alone.

Carrying your child in the post-partum period is important. As we have seen in previous chapters, these early weeks are vital for bonding and attachment, providing continuity and security, promoting breastfeeding and helping to reduce depression. So yes, we should carry our babies after birth. This doesn't need a sling; parents can hold their babies while sitting down and while reclining just as much as while they stand and walk around; it is the closeness, and the skin-to-skin that matter.

'Using a sling with my second child from the first day has changed everything from the first time around, mainly for my mental state. It's giving me that confirmation that I can still be present with my older babe and carry on with our life together, and the bond, oh my, the bond!' Beckah

Carrying a newborn baby can be very healing if birth has been traumatic or there has been previous loss.

'I had a tiny baby (4lb 5oz) and experienced a traumatic birth, I suffered with PTSD. At times this meant I was very anxious and wanted to keep my baby close to me to be sure she was safe. I started with a stretchy wrap when Poppy was just three weeks old. I truly believe babywearing strengthened my attachment with her and helped me to cope every day. I still carry my now toddler in a full buckle and hope to continue for as long as possible.' Jessica

There are garments that can be worn in hospital or in the early weeks after birth, mimicking the practice of putting a tiny newborn down the front of a shirt. Some of these (known as skin-to-skin tops or kangaroo care clothing) are designed for keeping baby skin-to-skin with the parent while reclining, and are not hands-free. Others are a little more structured (at least two layers of stretchy fabric) and provide enough support for baby that a parent can be hands-free and walk around, similar to a stretchy wrap. These can be most useful in hospital environments for their coolness and simplicity.

Breast and bottle-feeding in the early weeks can cause back, neck and shoulder pain, as can prolonged periods of one-sided carrying (which can also affect the pelvic floor and the symphysis pubis.) Being alert to the body's signals of discomfort and acting on them to frequently redistribute the strain is of great benefit in building up tolerance and strength.

As women recover their strength and are able to do more each day, their mobile carrying abilities increase. As women's bodies settle after pregnancy, with appropriate pelvic floor toning and correction of posture and alignment, carrying will become easier. Furthermore, as baby gets bigger and heavier, the parent's muscles will adapt to the gradually increasing weight and become more toned.

> '*Much of my pre-pregnancy life was spent in the mountains, and carrying my babies after their birth helped me get back in touch with my "home". It enabled me to very gradually and gently regain some fitness away from busy streets, and felt like less strain on the scar area than pushing a double buggy uphill.*' Carissa

Keeping a baby's weight high, snug and central encourages loading across the large weight-bearing axes of the body, preventing strain on muscles, ligaments and the pelvic floor and avoiding abdominal pressure. Lifting a baby to the chest should be done carefully, with knees bent and upright posture maintained, and pelvic floor and abdominal muscles engaged. Most types of carriers can be used after a vaginal birth.

Carrying after a caesarean is also possible, and there is an argument that it is even more important than after a vaginal delivery. As soon as surgery is over, a well baby can be given to its mother and skin-to-skin can begin. This is vitally important after a section, especially if it was an emergency and traumatic, which interrupts many of the biofeedback mechanisms involved in bonding. It is also important if the section was planned and baby was delivered before the biological hormone cascades of labour and birth were able to begin.

Women who did not have the birth experience they wished for may feel robbed and deprived of an important part of their baby's arrival. The subsequent feelings of sadness and grief, disappointment, or that they have let themselves or their baby down somehow, can significantly hamper the forming of attachment bonds and play a part in later postnatal depression. Mothers who experience this are very likely to find skin-to-skin contact and carrying extremely useful. The process of initiating and maintaining contact and loving touch often acts as a catalyst for oxytocin release, and this positive feedback mechanism encourages loving feelings to develop despite a less than 'perfect' start.

Once a mother is ready to move around and carry her child in her arms she can begin; she will be advised to carry nothing heavier than her baby. Some women choose to use slings immediately (especially if they are already familiar with slings and feel confident), while others will want to wait. If the mother is confined to hospital and alone for parts of the day, she may find a sling will help her to feel safer than carrying her baby loose in arms while she is still a little unsteady.

> 'Having a sling for carrying was very useful, as it was much easier and less painful than carrying in arms (less stress on abdominal muscles). It was great for bonding, especially since we were having trouble with breastfeeding.' Rebecca

> 'Carrying after my section helped me regain some of my emotional strength and feelings that I was a capable mother. It also gave me freedom to start going out when I couldn't drive and there was snow everywhere.' Lorette

The key factor is to avoid putting pressure on the abdomen or irritating the wound. Double-layer kangaroo-care shirts, or other soft carriers such as stretchy or woven wraps, high-carrying waistband-less carriers and ring slings in frontal tummy-to-tummy carries may be options to consider. Baby's legs should ideally be tucked into the M-shape, and this will also help to avoid feet kicking against a still-tender wound. As the scar heals, carriers with more structured waistbands will become more accessible.

Carrying in the post-partum period can actually help promote recovery. Holding a baby close in the anatomically correct position, so that their weight is well distributed through the large weight-bearing axes, will tone muscles and improve posture better than pushing a pram, which requires a strong forward lean. Being able to go for gradually longer and longer walks with your baby in a soft and comfortable sling rebuilds strength and releases endorphins. Participating in post-natal recovery programmes can be useful, but combining carrying and exercise/dance is best done with caution, as not every provider will have adequate knowledge of post-natal recovery (pelvic floor and diastasis recti) or the rate and speed of each woman's individual recovery from birth. Many have no specialist knowledge about safe sling use or how to protect a baby from sudden shaking movements, or how to avoid overloading still-recovering tissues with the extra load of a child in a sling. Walking with a baby in the sling, ensuring good alignment and posture, and gradually increasing speed and duration, is often enough exercise in the early months.

Using a sling allows families to settle back into the normal rhythms of daily life.

'Slinging my youngest helped me to be closer with my eldest. At the park, I could be at the bottom of the slide

and not behind a pram. At home, my husband works shifts and I swear we would never have had any dinner on the table if it wasn't for having a sling to get through what was conveniently her "witching hour" right when I needed to cook!' Lucy

Older siblings are often uncertain about the new addition to the family and uneasy about their place in it; they may need extra reassurance. They may want to return to their mother's arms and be close to her body, to reinforce the attachment bond.

'During the intense post-birth bonding period with D I began to use a couple of wraps that had been favourites of R, the new big brother. It almost felt like a betrayal! But one afternoon, R asked if he could come up for a front carry in his favourite wrap, something he hadn't done for ages, and we twirled round the lounge together laughing while my husband cuddled the new baby. I think that was a really healing moment for us and let my eldest know he still had an important place in my arms too.' Emma

Toddlers who want to be carried after birth present more of a challenge, especially if the pelvic floor is weak and there is diastasis recti. Many specialists suggest waiting until these issues have resolved and the mother is functionally strong before beginning to carry toddlers again; how long this takes will vary widely. Seated cuddles are always good! Generally, mothers who are well used to carrying toddlers will find it easier to resume carrying than those beginning for the first time, and front carrying may be the most suitable position (rather than hip or back carries) to avoid straining still-healing tissue. The post-partum period may therefore be a great opportunity for other caregivers in the family to share the carrying.

'Carrying our eldest son (3) enabled my wife to give her attention to our new baby. It gave us much needed daddy and son bonding, at a time when he was feeling insecure with the arrival of the new baby.' Mal

Carrying in pregnancy

Many mothers wonder if they can safely continue to carry their children while pregnant with a new baby. Having established a close bond and chosen a carrier for comfort and practicality, they are keen to continue to meet their child's needs for contact.

'I knew that I needed to make the most of carrying my girl before her sibling was born as things were about to change for all of us. She needed me too, so I carried her as long as I could during my pregnancy. Her weight balanced out my bump and actually made my back pain more manageable by being corrective.' Jody

Other mothers may not have a choice, especially if there will be a small age gap between siblings and the older child is not yet walking reliably, or if he becomes worried by the impending changes to the family structure and needs extra closeness and reassurance.

'My little girl is very strong-willed so if she wanted up for a carry while I was pregnant, it was simply the path of least resistance. There were a few times when she was poorly, others when she was tired or I simply had things to do. It was all about practicality and doing whatever made my day a bit easier.' Lindsay

It is worth reflecting on the fact that women around the world have, for many generations past, carried older children on their bodies while pregnant, so it is certainly possible. In societies where babywearing is a part of everyday life, child-carrying is traditionally shared in large families, with older siblings carrying younger ones, or close family members taking their turn. Women in more Westernised societies may feel more isolated and unsupported, and may need to carry their own children for longer periods and more often than in traditional societies.

Babywearing in pregnancy is possible for the majority of women if they are in good health and there is no medical reason to avoid lifting loads. Those who are already used to carrying toddlers will find it simple to continue; their body strength and tolerance has grown with their child's weight and little may need to change until the bump is large.

> '*We needed to walk the dog and I wanted to be able to go to the dog trials and carrying was much more convenient than a buggy. My body was used to carrying, so we just carried on!*' Lucy

Those who are new to carrying (and looking for a solution for an uncertain or distressed older child) may find it more of a challenge, just as if they had a new job which required sudden frequent heavy lifting. In these circumstances, it would be wise to get some support from your local sling professionals to find out which slings will work best for you and be comfortable. Once equipped with an appropriate sling, it is wise to stick to carrying for short periods and gradually increase the duration of use.

First trimester

The maternal body undergoes changes during pregnancy that can have an impact on the type of carrying women find comfortable. In the first trimester, symptoms such as nausea or lower abdominal discomfort can affect how much a woman feels able to carry; pressure around the stomach can feel intolerable. Fatigue and low back pain can take their toll as well, and changes in blood volume can cause lightheadedness or dizziness. Such symptoms may make carrying children uncomfortable or even inadvisable, and medical advice should be sought and respected. It is important for women to listen to what their bodies need and be responsive; this may mean changing which carrier they are using, changing position frequently, or even not carrying at all for a while.

All being well, however, most carriers can be used in early pregnancy. There is no need to fear that the growing baby will be squashed by waistbands, for example. On the whole, the carrier that a mother has been using until she discovered she was pregnant is fine while the foetus's body is still small and mostly contained within the pelvic brim. Front carries, hip and back carries are all appropriate.

This may be a good time to begin learning new carries or investigating other slings to accommodate a growing bump. At this stage the toddler's weight is still being distributed around the mother's body and it is not resting on the bump, so it is an opportunity to initiate change while still enjoying front carries.

If there is any discomfort from abdominal pressure, altering the type of carry can be very useful. Front carries that don't use a waistband and hip and back carries help to avoid any central abdominal pressure. Mei tais (and their variants) and woven wraps offer high back carries, and can be tied in ways that have no knots around the middle at all (for example, 'tying Tibetan'). A carrier with a waistband could be moved low down to settle around the hips (as long as the carried child remains snug and close enough to kiss, with an uncompromised airway), or moved higher up nearer the ribs.

Second trimester

As the growing bump begins to have an impact on a mother's shape, moving to hip or back carries may feel much more comfortable. Front carrying may become awkward as the child will be very high, and it is best to avoid a heavy toddler's weight sitting on top of a bump.

Hip carrying (with adjustable buckle carriers, mei tais, ring slings, other one-shouldered carriers or wraps) can become a fantastically useful option for quick up-and-downs; many parents carry toddlers loose in arms on their hips in daily life (usually with frequent changes of position and for short durations). A sling can add a little support if used well, but it does not mimic in-arms carrying as most of the weight of the child is borne by a single shoulder rather than the spine and lower body. It is very common for people to find themselves misaligned with hip carries, leaning away from the side the child is sitting on, finding their shoulders and upper body rotated, and experiencing a lot of pulling strain on the ring-shoulder. Trying to fit a big toddler on the hip in a very lateral position (to avoid sitting on a bump) may also mean that the shoulders are out of alignment, as one shoulder has to be held behind the central plane to fit around the child's body, putting a rotatory torsion on the spine.

Those who love ring slings and other hip carriers have often already learned how to minimise these alignment issues. It is worth being aware that prolonged hip carrying in pregnancy may also have an impact on the pelvis and its stability, especially as ligaments begin to soften and loosen in preparation for birth. If you begin to experience any discomfort with carrying then it is sensible to check your posture to make sure your spine is not twisting. Try frequent switching of sides, reduce the duration of carrying, and see your local specialist for support.

Back carrying is a good solution for many; there is more space on the back for a bigger child, enabling close contact without putting any pressure on the bump. The maternal body may be able to balance the front and back loads better with a more equal pull on the weight-bearing axes, but as the load grows, the strain will increase and some women will choose to stop carrying sooner than others, or reduce the duration of sling use. The carrier on the back should be used in such a way that the child is held snugly and as close as possible to the mother's centre of gravity, and needs to fit well to help with weight distribution. The core muscles of the abdomen and lower back/buttocks, as well as the joints of the spine and hips and knees, are having to work harder than usual; any pain or soreness during carrying, or stiffness and aching afterwards, should encourage a woman to assess whether it is appropriate to continue. Asking a sling and carrier consultant for help may be very useful.

Logistically, waistbands may begin to become difficult to fit above the bump and may no longer be supportive due to the changing angle of the band and how it functions when distributing weight around the pelvis. It is up to the individual to decide when the waistband is no longer the best option. At this stage, carriers with soft waistbands that will mould around the mother's shape, or no waistband at all, may be more useful. These wraparound carriers focus mainly on binding a child's body as close to his mother's as possible, for example mei tais, onbuhimos and podaegis, as well as woven wraps. These can be tied gently above the bump, or spread around the chest and shoulders, putting the weight much more on the mother's upper body. Learning how to do this well and comfortably may need practice and building up of strength due to the new position.

Third trimester

In this last part of pregnancy, the maternal body is carrying a significant extra load; movement may feel more cumbersome and the mother may not want to carry any more than she has to.

Furthermore, the levels of relaxin increase significantly; ligaments and tendons soften and become more elastic. This helps the pelvic outlet to widen ready for delivery and also loosens and softens the intercostal muscles and ligaments between the ribs to allow expansion of the chest. These changes all affect load-bearing and every pregnant mother will vary in what she feels able to do; each successive pregnancy also affects carrying ability.

In the third trimester, high, supportive back carries with soft slings tend to work best; woven wraps in multiple layer carries or supportive single layers are useful, as are mei tais and their variants, all of which keep toddler weight high, snug and central, minimising any uneven pressure on the pelvis and spine and also balancing out the weight of the bump. Carrying may be only for short periods, and hip carries are best kept to a minimum.

Once the baby has been born, the maternal body will take time to recover. It may be some time before a mother feels well and strong enough to begin carrying her toddler again; the pelvic floor and stretched abdominal muscles need time to tone and strengthen. For this reason, many experienced professionals advise that post-partum women carry only their newborn for the first few weeks and months, then begin to carry their toddler again in front carries before they consider restarting back carrying. Methods for getting a heavy toddler on the back will need to be considered; swinging and scooting methods may place inappropriate strain on still-recovering ligaments and muscles. This will of course depend on individual circumstances; back carrying may be preferable to pushing heavy buggies! Tandem carries may be necessary from an early stage, and it would be wise to visit your local sling professional to get some support with carrying two children if you are not experienced.

> *'I don't drive, and I remember my father-in-law seeing me tandem carry my toddler and the new baby for the*

first time. He was shocked and concerned. I laughed and said, 'but I've been doing this for ages, until the day he was born! He's just gone from being carried down there to being carried up here!' Mel

Carrying older children

'I wish I had known about slings when I had my first child!' Izzy

'My son suddenly wants to be carried all the time and he's so heavy now, I feel like we missed the boat.' Tara

Do these comments seem familiar? I hear this kind of thing almost daily, and while part of me rejoices that these parents now know how fantastic slings can be, I appreciate their sadness at what they feel they missed.

But big kids need to be carried too. How many of us have hoicked our hefty toddlers onto our hips when their legs get tired, or felt little arms wind around our necks when they are tearful? How many of our huge preschoolers still appreciate long hugs and piggyback rides? All children need closeness, long beyond the baby stage, long after they take their first steps, long after they start school... and so do grown-ups! Loving contact is vital to our emotional health, from cradle to grave.

Let's look at some reasons why some older children may want to be carried beyond the baby stage.

A sling is, at its most basic, a tool for enabling close contact, almost like another pair of enfolding arms, while your real arms can be used for other things. A good sling, when used well, provides a feeling of all-around gentle pressure, as if being hugged all over. This can be very valuable for children struggling with sadness, sensory overload, tiredness or fear from loud noises. Being close to a parent's body is reassuring and sends a valuable message to a child: 'You are loved. I will look after you when you are unhappy, I will keep you close when you need it. I am always here for you.'

> *'Now my little man is walking (and running) he is so busy with his important baby business and I'm able to do much more around the house compared to when he was permanently attached to me as a newborn. I suddenly noticed that we weren't spending the time together that we used to and I missed it. At seventeen months, carrying him is even more special as I no longer take it for granted that it will last forever because it no longer happens every day. It allows us to reconnect and share each other in a way that we couldn't before. Even seemingly mundane tasks like the weekly shop are precious as we rekindle our closeness.'* Rachel

Sometimes, after a traumatic experience such as feeling lost, or getting hurt, a child will ask for a cuddle. An unwell child often just wants to be close to someone who loves him. A child who is overtired or overwrought may find it hard to switch off or wind down and the calming influence of an adult's supportive love can allow them to relax.

> *'Carrying my older ones allowed me to retain that closeness and contact when it was needed. Although their legs were more than strong enough to carry them, there were times when they were just too tired, out of sorts, were ill or had hurt themselves, or when they simply needed to be close to me for a while! I can't count the number of times a tantrum was approaching for one of the aforementioned reasons, when getting them to snuggle on my back just*

dissolved all the hurt and upset and left us both feeling closer and calmer. I can't imagine a more loving way to respond to my children's needs.' Lucy

Slings can be very useful in busy or group situations where a walking child could get overwhelmed or lost.

'My sling is a valuable practical tool, especially for my two-year-old toddler. We don't drive so we rely on public transport to get around and our highly mobile little boy loves to walk, but on the odd occasion where it isn't safe or he could get lost (like in a busy Christmas Eve train station or around an airport) a sling is invaluable. I really think he enjoys these moments of calm in his busy little life and it means that we can navigate more challenging situations without needing to worry about him… and the ability to pin him down for a cuddle is also welcomed!' Lauren

A sling is as valid a means of transport as a pushchair, can be more convenient, and is far more comfortable than achingly weary in-arms carrying, or coaxing a tired child along. Some find it easier to manage than a heavy buggy.

'With two toddler boys, I needed to move on from pushing an empty double pram round in case they got tired. Slings gave us freedom; my boys could run and adventure as much as they wanted, and I always had the means to carry at least one of them should they get tired, fall or just need me.' Sharon

'It's so much easier to carry my children in slings than push a heavy double buggy. I don't have to plan my route to avoid steps like with the buggy, I have my hands free

to hold on to my eldest child's hand and my toddler gets to feel close to me like his baby sister. It's definitely less to worry about having both kids strapped on as I know exactly where they are and my toddler can't run off, but he's happy as he's high up, so can see more than he would walking or in the buggy.' Lauren

Carrying bigger kids is fun, when they want to be carried, and brings joy to parent and child, as well as greater freedom to explore.

'I carry my 2.5 year old because we can talk about all kinds of things, I think we have more conversations walking about using the carrier than we do in the house as she has my undivided attention and there's lots going on.' Merry

'I thoroughly enjoy still using the sling with my three-year-old as it enables us to do things that he might not manage all by himself, like climbing our local hills or hiking in the Peaks. We also use it as bonding time on the way to and from nursery which has always helped him with settling. Carrying an empty sling is a lot less annoying than pushing an empty buggy!' Jenny

'I carry my boy (26 months) to get stuff done safely out and about. He has always been a bit of a floor-treasure hunter and won't tolerate a pram, so it keeps him safe when he spots bottle tops in the road! It also means dog walks take as long as they should instead of 30 minutes to traverse the street, and he can see the river when we cross the bridge and spy into the allotments when we walk past them all. He's seen plenty – a fox he would have missed otherwise – plus getting the buggy to the best places would be a

challenge, and little legs tire often. My personal favourite, though, is hearing him sing softly as we travel.' Nat

Parents often find great comfort in their children's desire for closeness, and discover a whole new way to see the world. Families need to spend time together to be able to thrive as a whole, and carrying can be healing for parents.

'*I love carrying Noah who is 28 months, as it lets me see the world from his eyes. I see how magical discovering everything is for him, and rediscover many things myself. We are able to talk about what we are doing ('daddy, what do?'), or whatever he sees and wants to learn more about. He chooses the sling whenever he is getting overwhelmed to calm down and take a breather. It has also helped build our bond as I spent some of last year away from him working and he has had to adapt to being a big brother along with all the other trials and tribulations of being a two-year-old. Before we discovered carrying, I struggled in very busy places or at some social gatherings, but now with Noah in the sling I notice less about crowds and become less awkward socially.'* Mark

Some woodland kindergartens and nurseries with a strong outdoor focus have begun to use slings as a way to keep children warm and safe when needed.

'*At our woodland kindergarten carrying the children is invaluable. It gives children a place to rest but still feel included, it gives them comfort and warmth when outside all day away from their parents and it means our hands are free to play, interact and 'work' with the rest of the children. One day a child took a nap on a staff member's back; she led the children foraging for apples and blackberries.'* Helen

As we've discussed, carrying an older child in pregnancy can be an opportunity to help deepen relationships and prepare for the new arrival and can also help with sibling jealousy. Once baby is here, an older child who is feeling disconnected or displaced may really appreciate the reassurance that comes from being cuddled or carried. Sometimes tandem carrying (both children at once) is possible and can be very useful.

> 'Carrying two doesn't happen very regularly as my eldest is five but being able to say yes when he asks has helped immensely in reassuring him that his place in my heart and in my sling is still his. It has also helped my two to develop a caring and fun relationship as we are always sharing giggles when tandem carrying.' Lorette

You can use pretty much any kind of sling with a bigger child, even a stretchy if it is a high-quality hybrid one. They tend to work best and most easily in front carries. Ring slings can also be fantastic, if you have the shoulder style that suits you best made of a fabric that is supportive enough. People often suggest linen or hemp or silk to add strength to the softness of cotton, but many 100 per cent cottons are more than sturdy enough for heavy children, who can become easier to carry as they develop more core strength. Older children help you to carry them, by actively clinging on rather than passively being manoeuvred, and will often want to get down again fairly quickly.

Woven wraps are the most versatile, as they can be tied in different ways, in different positions and with different levels of support. As with ring slings, the fabric used can make a difference to how a wrap feels – fibres with extra support can be helpful but may not be necessary, and, as above, understanding tightening techniques and how to get a good position can really help you make the most of your wrap.

You can get toddler-size mei tais, half-buckles and full-buckle carriers, even some up to preschool size. It is worth trying a few at your local sling library as one size does not fit all, and the body size and shape of the carrying parent plays a part too. (Some preschooler carriers will be too big in their shaping for petite mums, for example.) Waistbands may need to be worn lower (around the hips) for front carries, and some creative methods for getting a good seat in a back carry may be needed! Your local sling professionals will be able to see whether you really need a bigger carrier for your child; it may be that your current carrier, with just a few tweaks in technique, is fine. Many people upgrade to toddler carriers earlier than really necessary, or choose to buy a toddler carrier for their baby so that it will last longer, but a carrier that is too big for a child may be more problematic than one that is slightly small. If the panel is too big, the child won't be well supported and can slump down inside, the child may not be able to see properly, which may irritate them, and an over-wide carrier can put strain on over-stretched ligaments. Some carriers, however, are designed to grow with children.

Parents who carry older children in slings may well hear unwelcome comments such as 'He's too big to be carried like that, he'll never learn to walk!' or 'You'll just make that child clingy and spoil him' or even 'Only babies get carried.'

Unfortunately this is unsurprising, as slings are no longer a common sight in our culture, compared to pushchairs or push-along sit-on toys. Older children who can walk but are still carried in slings are even more unusual than babies in slings; strangely there seems to be much less of a reaction to older children enjoying piggybacks or shoulder and hip carrying, or to parents who use pushchairs with older children. Hopefully as the benefits of carrying into toddlerhood and beyond become better understood, society will start to change to be more supportive of parents choosing to meet their children's needs in this way.

Don't be afraid to carry your toddler; for every critical remark you get, you may have planted an idea about carrying in someone else's head. Ensure that your child doesn't feel hurt by any comments he overhears: sometimes talking about any incidents together afterwards can be helpful. Using a sling for your bigger child from time to time will not harm them, nor will it make them into babies again, any more than a hug or a hip carry would do. Having their needs met will add to their self-confidence and improve their ability to handle life later on.

Carrying two children

Sometimes parents need to carry two children at the same time; for example, a pre-walker and a new baby. This is often easier for those who have already carried their older child and have some skills already. Carrying the small one on the front in something like a wrap and the bigger child on the back in a buckle carrier is one way that can work well, or you can use two buckle carriers. Such carries are much more comfortable than they may sound on paper, because the weight is balanced (typically, bigger child is on the back) fairly evenly and muscles soon grow strong. If a mother has been carrying throughout pregnancy, her body will have been adjusting and toning with the gradually increasing load of one child on the outside and one growing inside. After birth, the bump simply moves up to be carried on the outside (with the usual caveat about ensuring sufficient post-natal recovery).

'Tandem carrying was a lifesaver with my middle children. I hadn't yet learned to drive, so I walked everywhere. With a 22-month age gap, tandem carrying was an inevitable part of life. My older son gradually walked more as the

months went by, but would still need a nap – tandeming meant I didn't have to schedule life around his nap. He was still my baby too, and needed the closeness babywearing brings. It was also a lovely way for him to bond with his little brother – I would regularly feel his hand come round to hold or stroke baby's foot in the summer months.' Mel

Slings can be absolutely vital for parents of twins. Having a child in each arm can leave you with no hands free to be able to do anything else. Carrying twins is especially hard work; double the load from the beginning, which is different from a parent who is used to carrying a toddler adding a new baby on the front. There are some carriers that are designed to carry two babies at once very simply, which is very useful as it can be hard to learn complex carrying skills with two young babies, though many do manage it with determination and support from local sling professionals.

'For me, carrying twins in my twin buckle carrier is all about the practicalities and I wouldn't be without it. I see twin mums struggling with heavy car seats and there are so many places a double buggy doesn't fit... with my sling, my hands are free, my twins are safe and I have the freedom to go anywhere. It's so needed for even the simple things that mums of one baby probably aren't aware of, such as getting from your car in the car park and into a building. Two babies get very heavy in your arms and leave you with no hand free to open the door, so even for really short trips the sling is invaluable. With my handbag items in the pocket of my front carrier and a change bag in the pocket of the back one, I feel like life is full of possibilities again and I'm not weighed down by the logistics of being a mum to multiples. Plus, what's

not to love about being a "mummy sandwich"!' Gilly
'Carrying my twins in my sling has given me some very precious bonding time and cuddles that aren't always possible in a hectic day in our lives!' Carissa

'Having twins often means you don't get as much "quality bonding" time or time for cuddles, skin-to-skin or just sitting interacting or communicating with each child. Carrying both of them in tandem is a heart-enriching way of fostering closeness physically and emotionally and having a rare moment of calm, all three of you at the same time, in an otherwise chaotic frenetic life!' Alex

Carrying unwell children or those with disabilities

Sick children will benefit from being carried just as much as any other child, and more so, if they are afraid or in pain. Airway safety is of prime importance. Care and consideration will be needed for working around practical issues like oxygen or feeding tubes, surgical wounds or plaster casts. Babies in bar and boots or harnesses for situations like talipes (club foot) or hip dysplasia can be carried too, with support. Children with problems of prematurity, developmental delay or complex illnesses can usually be carried safely, with expert guidance. Please do go and see your local sling consultant, and ask your doctors for advice about how your child should be handled. Many medical staff may not have a wide experience of slings and showing them what you are hoping to use can be very useful to add to their knowledge and perhaps encourage them to consider advising carriers for the next little patient they have. Any child who can be carried in arms can usually be carried in a sling with the right support.

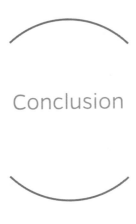

Conclusion

Our modern society is highly pressurised and artificial. We live under electric lights, we measure ourselves by clocks and deadlines, and we make choices based on societal expectations that are often more about productivity and achievement than our own health and wellbeing. Our children can become victims of this culture, being expected to fit into our lives and to grow up sooner than is biologically normal.

The early months and years of our babies' lives often set the scene for their whole future. A child's early experiences and the laying down of unconscious memories play a huge part in the development of their neurobiology. Neural pathways of behaviour are established, and the building of a set of strong, securely attached relationships is the cornerstone of emotional health. Love is vital to healthy lives, and close contact is necessary for children to thrive.

As we learn more about the way mothers' and babies' bodies actually work and fit together (the natural birth process, the size of babies' stomachs, their natural sleep patterns, the effect of cortisol on the growing brain, the power of oxytocin in forming attachments, the shape of maternal iliac crests for hip carrying), parents are beginning to change the way they bring up their children. They are turning to a more instinctive, responsive way of parenting. This is time-consuming and counter-cultural, and perceived as 'new-fangled', even though responsive parenting is as old as humanity itself.

What I've tried to show in this book is that carrying matters, for children, for parents, for society. Babywearing can meet so many needs, even in our modern world. It is a traditional practice that has stood the test of time, but its ongoing value is supported by modern scientific research. It is a simple way to foster a connection between parents and their children, to everyone's benefit. I hope that as more research emerges babywearing will come to be seen as an important public health measure, as well as a joyful personal experience.

Parenting is hard work and nobody ever gets it perfectly right. More often than not, however, the answers to the stresses and anxieties of family life can be found in the circle of strong arms and in a child's trusting response to the love that forms the bedrock of their world. What matters is the journey to creating a strong foundation that will become the springboard into a full and well-lived life. The path may be long and rocky, but our children give us the gift of parenthood, and when we carry them we give them the gift of ourselves.

'In a world which insists on moving at a pace that even most adults are challenged to keep up with, never mind our precious children, babywearing eases it all and steadies the world for both of us. The fast becomes slow, the chaos becomes calm, the loud becomes muffled; we are left with the sound of heartbeats, the rhythms of breathing and the sound of a kiss on the forehead.

Babywearing, for me, is sanctuary, intimacy and a peace that my son, myself, and this world needs.' Ricardo

Local help and support

There is a bewildering range of slings to choose from, so just like a book library, a *sling library* is a collection of slings and carriers that can be browsed, tried on (often with realistic weighted dolls) and taken away on hire to use at home.

Sling librarians usually have some form of peer supporter training in babywearing safety and will be able to help you find the right kind of carrier. Sling library sessions take place in people's homes, children's centres, church halls, cafes, theatres, supermarkets and so on. There is usually a small charge for the service as, unlike book libraries, which are publicly owned and funded by taxpayers, with paid staff, most sling libraries are run by committed volunteers, who often begin by buying slings with their own money, because they are enthusiastic babywearers and want to help others. The hire fees are essential to keep the service running, to replace worn-out carriers and add new ones, to pay rent for the rooms where sessions are held, and to pay for training, insurance, childcare and so on.

A sling and carrier consultant will have done further training, attending courses that are often three or four days long. They are teachers and have a greater depth of knowledge and expertise than peer supporters. Many run library sessions as well as more personal services such as small-group workshops, antenatal classes or one-to-one teaching sessions. Like peer supporters, consultants vary widely in experience and expertise.

A sling meet is a social event for parents who enjoy using carriers to get together. Some sling meets may have libraries or consultants in attendance, but the focus will be on friendship.

Find your local sling library, consultant or sling meet at www.slingpages.co.uk

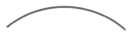

References

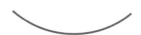

Introduction

1. Bowlby, J. Attachment and loss: Vol. 1. *Attachment* (2nd ed.). New York: Basic Books; 1969.
2. Ask Dr Sears *www.askdrsears.com*

Chapter 1

1. Kirkilionis, E. *A Baby Wants to Be Carried*. Pinter & Martin: London; 2014. p.22.
2. DeSilva JM, Lesnik JJ. Brain size at birth throughout human evolution: a new method for estimating neonatal brain size in hominins. *Journal of Human Evolution*. 2008; 55(6): 1064-74.
3. Wittman AB, Wall LL. The evolutionary origins of obstructed labor: bipedalism, encephalization, and the human obstetric dilemma. *Obstetrical & Gynecological Survey*. 2007; 62(11): 739.
4. Dunsworth HM, Warrener AG, Deacon T, Ellison PT, Pontzer H. Metabolic hypothesis for human altriciality. *Proceedings of the National Academy of Sciences*. 2012; 109(38):15212.
5. Holland D et al. Structural growth trajectories and rates of change in the first 3 months of infant brain development. *JAMA Neurology*. 2014; 71(10):s1266-1274.
6. Trevathan, WR. *Human Birth: An Evolutionary Perspective*. Aldine Transaction: New Jersey; 2011.

7. Berk LE. *Child Development* (8th ed.) Pearson: USA; 2009.

8. Kirkilionis E. *A Baby Wants to Be Carried*. Pinter & Martin: London; 2014.

9. Graham SM, Manara J, Chokotho L, Harrison WJ. Back-carrying infants to prevent developmental hip dysplasia and its sequelae: is a new public health initiative needed?' *Journal of Pediatric Orthopaedics*. 2015; Jan;35(1):57-61.

10. Wall-Scheffler CM, Geiger, K, Steudel-Numbers KL. Infant carrying: the role of increased locomotory costs in early tool development. *American Journal of Physical Anthropology*. 2007 Jun;133(2):841-6.

11. New Humanist *https://newhumanist.org.uk/2330/slings-arrows*

12. Blaffer H. *Mother Nature: Maternal instincts and the shaping of the species*. Vintage: London; 2000.

13. Lozoff B, Brittenham G. Infant care: cache or carry. *Journal of Pediatrics*. 1979; Sep;95(3):478-83.

14. Curtis, E. *The North American Indian*. Archive at the American Library of Congress.

Chapter 2

1. Heller, S. *Vital Touch: How Intimate Contact with Your Baby Leads to Happier, Healthier Development*. Henry Holt & Company: New York; 1997.

2. Esposito G et al. Infant calming responses during maternal carrying in humans and mice. *Current Biology*. 2013; May; 23(9):739–745.

3. Simply Psychology *http://www.simplypsychology.org/maslow.html*

4. Pollak SD et al. Neurodevelopmental effects of early deprivation in post-institutionalized children. *Child Development*. 2010; Jan-Feb; 81(1):224–236.

5. Gerhardt S. *Why Love Matters: How Affection Shapes a Baby's Brain*. Routledge: New York; 2004.

6. Shonkoff et al. Neuroscience, molecular biology, and the childhood roots of health disparities: building a new framework for health promotion and disease prevention. *JAMA*. 2009; 301(21):2252-9.

7. Gerhardt, op.cit.

8. Varendi H et al. Soothing effect of amniotic fluid smell in newborn infants. *Early Human Development*. 1998; Apr;51(1):47-55.

9. ICEA *http://icea.org/sites/default/files/Skin%20to%20Skin%20 Contact%20PP-FINAL.pdf*

10. Anderson GC. Current knowledge about skin-to-skin (kangaroo) care for

preterm infants. *Journal of Perinatology*. 1991; Sep;11(3):216-26.

11. Cochrane *http://www.cochrane.org/CD003519/PREG_early-skin-to-skin-contact-for-mothers-and-their-healthy-newborn-infants*

12. Lawn JE et al. Kangaroo mother care to prevent neonatal deaths due to preterm birth complications. *International Journal of Epidemiology*. 2010;39: i144–i154 *http://ije.oxfordjournals.org/content/39/suppl_1/i144.full.pdf+html*

13. National Institute for Clinical Excellence – Care of Women and their Babies

14. Bigelow A, Power M, MacLellan-Peters J, Alex M, McDonald C. Effect of mother/infant skin-to-skin contact on postpartum depressive symptoms and maternal physiological stress. *Journal of Obstetric Gynecologic and Neonatal Nursing*. 2012; May-Jun;41(3): 369-82. doi: 10.1111/j.1552-6909.2012.01350.x. Epub 2012 Apr 26.

15. Bowlby, op.cit., p.194.

16. Ainsworth MDS, Bell SM, Stayton DJ. Individual differences in the development of some attachment behaviors. *Merrill-Palmer Quarterly, Behavior and Development*. 1972; 18:123–143.

17. Stayton D, Ainsworth MDS. Development of separation behavior in the first year of life. *Developmental Psychology*. 1973;9:226- 235.

18. Salter MD, Ainsworth MDS, Bell SM. Attachment, exploration, and separation: illustrated by the behavior of one-year-olds in a strange situation. *Child Development*. 1970; Mar; 41(1):49-67. Available in *Evolutionary Psychology* ISSN 1474-7049. 2007; 5(1):140.

19. Rees CA. Thinking about children's attachments. *Archives of Disease in Childhood*. 2005; Oct; 90(10):1058-65.

20. Schön RA, Silvén M. Natural parenting – back to basics in infant care. *Evolutionary Psychology*. 2007; 5:102-183.

21. Prescott J. The origins of human love and violence. *Pre and Perinatal Psychology Journal*. 1996 Spring; 10(3):155.

22. Gerhardt, op.cit.

23. Tronick E, Adamson LB, Als H, and Brazelton TB. Infant emotions in normal and pertubated interactions. 1975. April; Paper presented at the biennial meeting of the Society for Research in Child Development, Denver, CO.

24. D'Antonio A. *Devouring Anxiety: Victorian Breastfeeding and the Modern Individual*. ProQuest: Ann Arbor; 2009.

25. Lozoff B and Brittenham G. Infant care: cache or carry. *The Journal of Pediatrics*. 1979; Sep; 95(3):478-83.

26. Hunziker UA, Barr RG. Increased carrying reduces infant crying: a

randomized controlled trial. *Pediatrics*. 1986; May; 77(5):641-8.

27. Baildam EM, Hillier VF, Menon S, Bannister RP, Bamford FN, Moore WMO and Ward BS. Attention to infants in the first year. *Child: Care, Health and Development*. 2000; 26:199–216.

28. Ainsworth, Bell and Stayton, op.cit., 1972.

29. Dettwyler K. 'A time to wean: The hominid blueprint for the natural age of weaning in modern human populations' in Stewart-MacAdam, P, Dettwyler, KA (eds). *Breastfeeding: Biocultural Perspectives*. Aldine deGruyter: New York; 1995.

30. Bowman K. *Move your DNA: Restore Your Health Through Natural Movement*. Propriometrics Press: Carlsborg; 2014.

31. Kerns KA et al. Mother-child attachment in later middle childhood: assessment approaches and associations with mood and emotion regulation. *Attachment & Human Development*. 2007; 9(1):33-53.

Chapter 3

1. Lawn JE et al, op.cit.

2. *Kangaroo Mother Care: a Practical Guide*. WHO: Geneva; 2003.

3. Anisfield E, Casper V, Nozyce M et al. Does infant carrying promote attachment? *Child Development*. 1990; 61(5):1617-1627.

4. Baronel L, Lionetti F. Attachment and emotional understanding: a study of late adopted pre-schoolers and their parents. *Child Care Health Development*. 2012; Sept; 38(5).

5. McCain G et al. Heart rate variability responses of a preterm infant to kangaroo care. *Journal of Obstetric Gynecologic and Neonatal Nursing*. 2005; 34(6):689-94.

6. Charpak N et al. Kangaroo mother care: 25 years after. *Acta Paediatrica*. 2005: 94(5):514-522.

7. Gregson S, Blacker J. Kangaroo care in pre-term or low birth weight babies in a postnatal ward. *British Journal of Midwifery*. 2011; 19:568–577.

8. Furman L. Correlates of lactation of very low birth weight infants. *Pediatrics*. 2002; 109(4):57.

9. Parker LA et al. Effect of early breast milk expression on milk volume and timing of lactogenesis stage II among mothers of very low birth weight infants: a pilot study. *Journal of Perinatology*. 2012; Mar;32(3):205-9.

10. Ludington-Hoe S. Breast infant temperature with twins during shared kangaroo care. *Journal of Obstetric, Gynecologic and Neonatal Nursing*. 2006; 35(2):223-231.

11. Eposito et al, op.cit.

12. Ferber et al. The effect of skin-to-skin contact (kangaroo care) shortly after birth on the neurobehavioral responses of the term newborn: a randomized, controlled trial. *Pediatrics*. 2004; 113:858-865.

13. Messmer P et al. Effect of kangaroo care on sleep time for neonates. *Pediatric Nursing*. 1997; 23(4):408-414.

14. Hunziker UA, Barr RG. Increased carrying reduces infant crying: a randomized controlled trial. *Pediatrics*. 1986; May; 77(5):641-8.

15. St James-Roberts I, Alvarez M, Csipke E, Abramsky T, Goodwin J and Sorgenfrei E. Infant crying and sleeping in London, Copenhagen and when parents adopt a 'proximal' form of care. *Pediatrics*. 2006; 117:e1146-e1155.

16. Kostandy et al. Kangaroo care (skin contact) reduces crying response to pain in preterm neonates: pilot results. *Pain Management Nursing*. 2008: 9:55-65.

17. Tasker A, Dettmar PW, Panetti M, Koufman JA, Birchall JP, and Pearson JP. Is gastric reflux a cause of otitis media with effusion in children? *The Laryngoscope*. 2002; 112:1930–1934.

18. Lawn et al, op.cit.

19. Turk AE, McCarthy JG, Thorne CH, Wisoff JH. The 'back to sleep campaign' and deformational plagiocephaly: is there cause for concern? *Journal of Craniofacial Surgery*. 1996; Jan;7(1):12-8.

20. Moore GA, Cohn JF, Campbell SB. Infant affective responses to mother's still face at 6 months differentially predict externalizing and internalizing behaviors at 18 months. *Developmental Psychology*. 2001; Sep;37(5):706-14.

Chapter 4

1. NICE guidelines [CG132]. Published date: November 2011.

2. Bick J, Dozier M. Mothers' and children's concentrations of oxytocin following close, physical interactions with biological and non-biological children'. *Developmental Psychobiology*. 2010; Jan; 52(1): 100–107.

3. Singh E. *The effects of various methods of infant carrying on the human body and locomotion*. A thesis submitted to the Faculty of the University of Delaware in partial fulfilment of the requirements for the degree of Honors Bachelor of Arts in Anthropology with Distinction, 2009.

Chapter 5

1. Stuebe A. The risks of not breastfeeding for mothers and infants. *Reviews in Obstetrics and Gynecology*. 2009; Fall; 2(4):222–231.

2. Washbrook E, Waldfogel J, Moullin S. Baby bonds, parenting,

attachment and a secure base for children. Sutton Trust. *http://www.suttontrust.com/researcharchive/baby-bonds/*

3. University of Notre Dame. 'Modern parenting may hinder brain development, research suggests'. *ScienceDaily*, 7 January 2013. *www.sciencedaily.com/releases/2013/01/130107110538.html*.

Chapter 6

1. Kornhauser Cerar L et al. A comparison of respiratory patterns in healthy term infants placed in car safety seats and beds. *Pediatrics*. 2009; Sept; 124(3).
2. Bass JL et al. The effect of chronic or intermittent hypoxia on cognition in childhood: a review of the evidence. *Pediatrics*. 2004; Sep; 114(3):805-816.
3. Stening W, Nitsch P, Wassmer G et al. Cardiorespiratory stability of premature and term infants carried in infant slings. *Pediatrics*. 2002;110(5):879-83.
4. Berk, Laura E. *Child Development* (8th ed.). Boston: Pearson; 2009.
5. Graham SM et al. Back-carrying infants to prevent developmental hip dysplasia and its sequelae: is a new public health initiative needed? *Journal of Pediatric Orthopaedics*. 2015; Jan; 35(1):57–61.

Chapter 8

1. The Royal College of Midwives. *Maternal Emotional Wellbeing and Infant Development* 2. November 2012.
2. Kornhauser Cerar L et al, op.cit.
3. Stening W, Nitsch P, Wassmer G et al, op.cit.

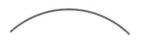

Further Reading and Resources

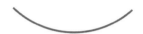

Bowman K. *Move your DNA: Restore Your Health through Natural Movement*. Lotus Publishing: Chichester; 2015.

Gerhardt S. *Why Love Matters: How affection shapes a baby's brain*. Routledge: New York; 2014.

Van Hout IC. *Beloved Burden: Babywearing Around The World*, KIT Publishers; 2011.

Kirkilionis E. *A Baby Wants to Be Carried*. Pinter & Martin, 2014.

The UP Project is a UK charity, whose mission is to ensure that children who are affected by disability, serious illness, depression, domestic abuse or poverty are given the opportunity to experience the benefits of being carried in a baby sling or carrier. www.theupproject.org.uk

Image Credits

p.13	Illustration by Jon Lander
p.69	Image licensed via Creative Commons: creativecommons.org/licenses/by-sa/3.0/legalcode
p.70	Image courtesy of Sheffield Sling Surgery
p.85	Image courtesy Lucy Davies
p.90	Image courtesy Juliette Daum, Baie Slings
p.95	Image courtesy Rosie Knowles
p.99	(L) Image courtesy Rosie Knowles
p.99	(R) Image courtesy Connecta Baby Ltd.
p.102	Image courtesy Rosie Knowles

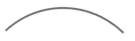

Acknowledgements

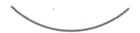

I would like to thank firstly, my husband Robert who has been my most loyal supporter and champion; our lives simply wouldn't work without him and his loving care. I thank our two children too, Fred and Maggie, who have shown us the power of close and loving contact, and I am grateful for their kindness in sharing their mother and their home with many other small children over the years. I like to feel I have a very large extended family and I am grateful to all these parents who have welcomed me into their lives and allowed me to support them in their journey of raising small people.

Over the last few years I have been blessed enough to work with and be encouraged by some fantastic people in the babywearing community who have been inspirational role models of integrity and dedication. I'm proud to call many of these people my friends, and their support has been of enormous value to me.

I would also like to thank my editor Susan who helped me enormously with the challenge of book writing, which is very different from magazine or website articles. I am grateful for her for giving me the chance to do this and for her patience as I fitted the writing into the crevices of a very busy life.

Lastly, I must thank the team of people working tirelessly with me in Sheffield at the Sling Surgery; I couldn't do it without them.

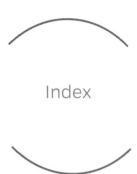

Index

The T.I.C.K.S. Rule for Safe Babywearing

Keep your baby close and keep your baby safe.
When you're wearing a sling or carrier, don't forget the **T.I.C.K.S.**

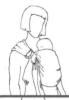

√ **TIGHT**

√ **IN VIEW AT ALL TIMES**

√ **CLOSE ENOUGH TO KISS**

√ **KEEP CHIN OFF THE CHEST**

√ **SUPPORTED BACK**

TIGHT – slings and carriers should be tight enough to hug your baby close to you as this will be most comfortable for you both. Any slack/loose fabric will allow your baby to slump down in the carrier which can hinder their breathing and pull on your back.

IN VIEW AT ALL TIMES – you should always be able to see your baby's face by simply glancing down. The fabric of a sling or carrier should not close around them so you have to open it to check on them. In a cradle position your baby should face upwards not be turned in towards your body.

CLOSE ENOUGH TO KISS – your baby's head should be as close to your chin as is comfortable. By tipping your head forward you should be able to kiss your baby on the head or forehead.

KEEP CHIN OFF THE CHEST – a baby should never be curled so their chin is forced onto their chest as this can restrict their breathing. Ensure there is always a space of at least a finger width under your baby's chin.

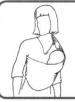

SUPPORTED BACK – in an upright carry a baby should be held comfortably close to the wearer so their back is supported in its natural position and their tummy and chest are against you. If a sling is too loose they can slump which can partially close their airway. (This can be tested by placing a hand on your baby's back and pressing gently - they should not uncurl or move closer to you.)

A baby in a cradle carry in a pouch or ring sling should be positioned carefully with their bottom in the deepest part so the sling does not fold them in half pressing their chin to their chest.